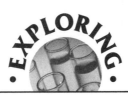

·EXPLORING·

SCIENCE AND MEDICAL DISCOVERIES

Medical Imaging

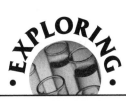

·EXPLORING·

SCIENCE AND MEDICAL DISCOVERIES

Medical Imaging

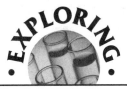

SCIENCE AND MEDICAL DISCOVERIES

Medical Imaging

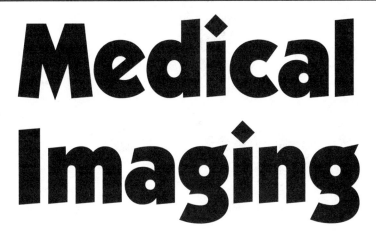

Clay Farris Naff, *Book Editor*

Bruce Glassman, *Vice President*
Bonnie Szumski, *Publisher*
Helen Cothran, *Managing Editor*
David M. Haugen, *Series Editor*

GREENHAVEN PRESS
An imprint of Thomson Gale, a part of The Thomson Corporation

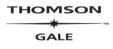

Detroit • New York • San Francisco • San Diego • New Haven, Conn.
Waterville, Maine • London • Munich

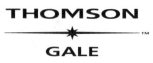

LIBRARY OF CONGRESS CATALOGING-IN-PUBLICATION DATA

Medical imaging / Clay Farris Naff, book editor.
    p. cm. — (Exploring science and medical discoveries)
Includes bibliographical references and index.
ISBN 0-7377-2829-9 (lib. : alk. paper)
    1. Diagnostic imaging. I. Naff, Clay Farris. II. Series.
RC78.7.D53M428   2006
616.07'54—dc22   2005046161

Printed in the United States of America

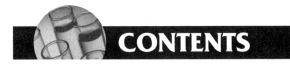

CONTENTS

Chapter 1: The Early History of Medical Imaging

1. Before Imaging: An Ancient Greek View of Anatomy

by Galen

An ancient Greek physician explains that his theories
pertaining to the human circulatory system and skeleton are based on studies of animal bodies and human
corpses that he comes across by chance.

2. Listening to the Body: A History of the Early Stethoscope

by D.M. Cammann

A nineteenth-century physician reviews the history of
the best diagnostic tool doctors had prior to the discovery of X-rays: the stethoscope.

3. The Discovery of X-Rays

by Neil Sclater

In 1895 German physics professor Wilhelm C. Röntgen accidentally discovered X-rays and how they could
be used to image the interior of the human body.

4. The Origins of Magnetic Resonance Imaging

by The Economist

Since its emergence in the 1970s, magnetic resonance
imaging, or MRI, has become one of the most useful
of medical imaging tools.

Chapter 2: Principal Types of Medical Imaging

1. Medical Imaging: An Overview of Techniques

Modern medicine draws on a wide array of imaging tools. Many of these tools employ X-rays, but others such as ultrasound and magnetic resonance are proving safer or superior for imaging certain parts of the body.

2. Conventional X-Rays and Radiation

Since their discovery in 1895, X-rays have become a widely used medical imaging procedure. Although X-rays produce harmful radiation, today's patients are not harmed by X-ray procedures.

3. Computed Tomography

A radiologist and a radiological specialist describe the great improvements in X-ray imaging made possible by computed tomography.

4. Magnetic Resonance Imaging

Using powerful magnets and radio waves, magnetic resonance imaging creates detailed images of the body's interior without the danger of radiation exposure.

5. Ultrasound

Ultrasound imagers emit high-frequency sound waves into a patient's body and capture the echoes, which can be turned into live-action images of the body's interior.

Chapter 3: Contemporary Issues in Medical Imaging

1. Mammography Is Unreliable

The utility of mammograms has been oversold. Early

detection of breast cancer through mammography does not result in less aggressive treatments, and unnecessary mastectomies through misdiagnosis are a common result of mammograms.

Chapter 4: Emerging Applications in Medical Imaging

capture more detail with less discomfort to the patient, and may eventually treat as well as detect breast cancer.

6. Computers Are Vital to New Imaging Techniques

A physicist describes how the use of computers has allowed for great improvements in medical imaging.

7. Wavelets Are Enhancing Medical Imaging

Three experts describe how wavelets, mathematical tools that help computers make data intelligible, are enhancing medical imaging technologies.

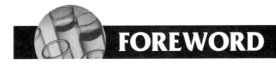

FOREWORD

Most great science and medical discoveries emerge slowly from the work of generations of scientists. In their laboratories, far removed from the public eye, scientists seek cures for human diseases, explore more efficient methods to feed the world's hungry, and develop technologies to improve quality of life. A scientist, trained in the scientific method, may spend his or her entire career doggedly pursuing a goal such as a cure for cancer or the invention of a new drug. In the pursuit of these goals, most scientists are single-minded, rarely thinking about the moral and ethical issues that might arise once their new ideas come into the public view. Indeed, it could be argued that scientific inquiry requires just that type of objectivity.

Moral and ethical assessments of scientific discoveries are quite often made by the unscientific—the public—sometimes for good, sometimes for ill. When a discovery is unveiled to society, intense scrutiny often ensues. The media report on it, politicians debate how it should be regulated, ethicists analyze its impact on society, authors vilify or glorify it, and the public struggles to determine whether the new development is friend or foe. Even without fully understanding the discovery or its potential impact, the public will often demand that further inquiry be stopped. Despite such negative reactions, however, scientists rarely quit their pursuits; they merely find ways around the roadblocks.

Embryonic stem cell research, for example, illustrates this tension between science and public response. Scientists engage in embryonic stem cell research in an effort to treat diseases such as Parkinson's and diabetes that are the result of cellular dysfunction. Embryonic stem cells can be derived from early-stage embryos, or blastocysts, and coaxed to form any kind of human cell or tissue. These can then be used to replace damaged or diseased tissues in those suffering from intractable diseases. Many researchers believe that the use of embryonic stem cells to treat human diseases promises to be one of the most important advancements in medicine.

However, embryonic stem cell experiments are highly controversial in the public sphere. At the center of the tumult is the fact that in order to create embryonic stem cell lines, human embryos must be destroyed. Blastocysts often come from fertilized eggs that are left over from fertility treatments. Critics argue that since blastocysts have the capacity to grow into human beings, they should be granted the full range of rights given to all humans, including the right not to be experimented on. These analysts contend, therefore, that destroying embryos is unethical. This argument received attention in the highest office of the United States. President George W. Bush agreed with the critics, and in August 2001 he announced that scientists using federal funds to conduct embryonic stem cell research would be restricted to using existing cell lines. He argued that limiting research to existing lines would prevent any new blastocysts from being destroyed for research.

Scientists have criticized Bush's decision, saying that restricting research to existing cell lines severely limits the number and types of experiments that can be conducted. Despite this considerable roadblock, however, scientists quickly set to work trying to figure out a way to continue their valuable research. Unsurprisingly, as the regulatory environment in the United States becomes restrictive, advancements occur elsewhere. A good example concerns the latest development in the field. On February 12, 2004, professor Hwang Yoon-Young of Hanyang University in Seoul, South Korea, announced that he was the first to clone a human embryo and then extract embryonic stem cells from it. Hwang's research means that scientists may no longer need to use blastocysts to perform stem cell research. Scientists around the world extol the achievement as a major step in treating human diseases.

The debate surrounding embryonic stem cell research illustrates the moral and ethical pressure that the public brings to bear on the scientific community. However, while nonexperts often criticize scientists for not considering the potential negative impact of their work, ironically the public's reaction against such discoveries can produce harmful results as well. For example, although the outcry against embryonic stem cell research in the United States has resulted in fewer embryos being destroyed, those with Parkinson's, such as actor Michael J. Fox, have argued that prohibiting the development of new stem cell lines ultimately will prevent a timely cure for the disease that is killing Fox and thousands of others.

Greenhaven Press's Exploring Science and Medical Discoveries series explores the public uproar that often follows the disclosure of scientific advances in fields such as stem cell research. Each anthology traces the history of one major scientific or medical discovery, investigates society's reaction to the breakthrough, and explores potential new applications and avenues of research. Primary sources provide readers with eyewitness accounts of crucial moments in the discovery process, and secondary sources offer historical perspectives on the scientific achievement and society's reaction to it. Volumes also contain useful research tools, including an introductory essay providing important context, and an annotated table of contents enabling students to quickly locate selections of interest. A thorough index helps readers locate content easily, a detailed chronology helps students trace the history of the discovery, and an extensive bibliography guides readers interested in pursuing further research.

Greenhaven Press's Exploring Science and Medical Discoveries series provides readers with inspiring accounts of how generations of scientists made the world's great discoveries possible and investigates the tremendous impact those innovations have had on the world.

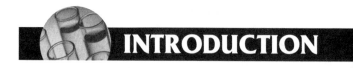

Medical Imaging: Boundless Vision, Staggering Costs

Imagine a visit to the doctor in the centuries before medical imaging became possible. Most physicians had very little knowledge about the interior of the human body. Surgeons got glimpses, to be sure, but they were occupied primarily with sewing up or cauterizing wounds and setting broken bones. More adventurous surgery was constrained by the tendency for fatal infection to follow (early doctors had no understanding of germs) and by severe laws, such as the ancient Code of Hammurabi, which specified that a surgeon's hands would be cut off if his patient died from the operation. Taboos against dissections also prevailed in much of the world. With only a skin-deep knowledge of the human body and its ailments, doctors often did more harm than good.

In medieval Europe, whatever a patient's ailment, the doctor would likely have treated him or her by trying to restore the balance of "humors"—blood, phlegm, black bile, and yellow bile—in the body. Relying on ancient Greek beliefs about medicine, European doctors assumed that all disease resulted from imbalances in the proportions of these supposed humors. During these times, doctors believed that bleeding patients would restore the balance of the humors. Needless to say, the cure was often worse than the disease.

In China doctors would also have attempted to restore harmony to the patient's body. However, they sought to balance not humors but a mysterious energy called chi. Ancient Chinese doctrines emphasized harmony and order, so anatomical drawings often portrayed the internal organs arranged symmetrically down the left and right sides of the body. To restore the balance of chi, practitioners of Chinese medicine employed a variety of treatments that included moxibustion, the burning of herbs directly on the skin.

Confusion About Organs

Ancient Egyptians, who practiced ritual dissection in the course of embalming, had a better opportunity than most to understand human anatomy. Nevertheless, physicians in this ancient civilization were guided by religious doctrines that led them to confuse the functions of the heart and brain. Some of them were convinced that the brain pumped blood, while the heart was widely considered the seat of thought and emotion. Since ancient Egyptian physicians occasionally attempted brain surgery, this misapprehension must have led to disastrous outcomes.

Even after an accurate understanding of anatomy began to emerge in Europe in the sixteenth century, treatments based on the four-humors theory predominated. Moreover, when it came to diagnosis, physicians still had to rely largely on external symptoms and guesswork. It did little good to know the location of the heart, for example, if the organ could not be examined for disease while the patient was alive. In case of accidents doctors could not even detect, let alone treat, minor bone fractures.

It was not until 1895, when Wilhelm C. Röntgen discovered X-rays, that physicians finally had a reliable diagnostic tool. His discovery launched the era of medical imaging. One of the first X-ray photographs the German physicist produced was of his wife's hand. The medical implications were immediately apparent. Within months the clinical use of X-rays to diagnose bone fractures was under way. In the United States inventor Thomas Edison began to manufacture X-ray devices.

Diagnoses Improve, but Costs Soar

Medical imaging has transformed modern medicine. Physicians no longer have to guess about the location and function of bones and organs to make their diagnoses. However, as medical imaging technology has improved, making diagnoses increasingly accurate, the rising costs of imaging procedures is leading to calls for a reduction in their use. Ironically, just as doctors have at their disposal the means for making the most accurate diagnoses in history, they are under increasing pressure not to exploit this advantage. Most of the concerns about cost came long after the discovery of X-rays. Indeed, X-rays were, and continue to be, quite economical.

For more than fifty years, X-ray imaging stood alone as an affordable and useful medical imaging technology. In addition to producing X-ray photographs, known as radiographs, Röntgen's discovery could be used in conjunction with a glowing screen to produce live images of internal structures. These devices, called fluoroscopes, were so inexpensive that many shoe stores installed them so that customers could see their toes wiggling inside shoes as they tried them on.

Eventually, however, it became evident that overexposure to X-rays carries significant risks. As early as 1904, deaths attributed to X-rays began to be recorded, but no one understood exactly why. As one historian notes, "Throughout these earliest years, as the obituaries of radiology pioneers appeared with somber regularity in the journals, researchers worked to untangle the paradox by which the new discovery could kill as well as cure."[1] It is now known that the high-energy radiation constituting X-rays easily damages DNA, leading to cell death and, sometimes years later, cancer.

The evident hazards of X-ray exposure, along with the limitations of the technology to image soft tissues, eventually inspired the development of other imaging techniques. Ultrasound, a nonradioactive alternative to X-rays, came into wide use in the 1960s. However, a genuine revolution began in the 1970s, when computers were harnessed to enhance medical imaging.

The Power of Computing

Conventional X-ray machines were transformed by a technique called tomography, meaning sectional imaging. Ordinarily, an X-ray image squashes everything between the source and the photographic plate into a single two-dimensional image. A hard object near the surface will mask anything beneath it. By taking multiple, narrowly focused X-ray images at various angles and processing them in a computer, radiologists are able to obtain a detailed "slice" image of internal structures without concern about masking effects. The slices can be combined into three-dimensional images. With the improvement in imaging, however, came a considerable increase in costs. As of 2005 the cost of a computed tomography (CT) scan was up to seven times that of a conventional X-ray.

The computer revolution also made possible magnetic resonance imaging (MRI). Combining data from huge and powerful magnets with pulses of radio waves, computers plot the location of trillions of hydrogen atoms within the body and transform the data into images. MRI is not just an alternative imaging system; it provides a whole new view. Since an MRI scanner can identify the type and location of any tissue anywhere in the body, it can be used to create a three-dimensional model as well as a two-dimensional image of any organ. A later version, called functional MRI, provides doctors with the ability to track the flow of blood through the heart or to capture images of the brain using glucose as fuel. Costly to build and expensive to operate, MRI machines nevertheless spread rapidly through the U.S. health-care system, from a handful in the early 1980s to more than twenty-five hundred two decades later. At roughly eight hundred dollars per image, MRI is even more costly than CT, but it is far from being the most costly of the new imaging technologies.

An even more expensive method of imaging has come into wide use: position-emission tomography, or PET. Patients are injected with a briefly radioactive substance that is absorbed by cancerous tissues. The unstable substance emits positrons, which give off a flash of photons when they encounter nearby electrons. These photons are detected by a scanner surrounding the patient. By plotting the trajectories of the photons, the PET scanner can produce a detailed image of the tumor even within hard-to-image locations such as the brain. At approximately two thousand dollars per scan, it ranks among the most expensive imaging techniques in medicine. In 1999 a pair of radiologists wrote in a professional journal about the future of the technology: "Although positron emission tomography (PET) is expensive in terms of absolute dollars per exam . . . its superior accuracy for multiple oncologic indications makes it a promising tool."[2] Along with CT and MRI, its usage continues to climb.

The Mammogram Debate

One of the greatest controversies over medical imaging and its costs arises from mammography. Breast cancer is a widespread and potentially fatal illness. Although both men and women can contract it, the disease primarily afflicts older women. Since the late 1970s women over the age of forty have been advised to have an annual mammogram—an X-ray examination of their breasts— to identify any cancerous growths as early as possible. The alternative, a manual exam for lumps, can also find tumors but only after they have grown to a palpable size.

A typical mammogram involves conventional X-ray equipment and costs less than $150. In the aggregate, however, mammograms have added tremendously to the nation's health-care costs. In Wisconsin, for example, a study showed that the number of annual mammograms grew by more than tenfold in a decade, leaping from 31,000 in 1980 to 383,000 in 1990.

The value of mammograms for premenopausal women has been much disputed. In 1997 a National Institutes of Health panel released a consensus paper concluding that "for women ages 40–49, during the first 7–10 years following initiation of screening, breast cancer mortality is no lower in women who were assigned to screening than in controls."[3] In other words, mammograms provided on average no benefit to women in this age group.

Nationwide, the bill for providing annual mammograms to women in that age range has been estimated as high as $2.5 billion—more than the budget of the National Cancer Institute. Additional costs follow from mammograms. About half the women who have regular mammograms are mistakenly told they have something wrong at some point. Tumors identified in such screenings often turn out, after biopsy or surgery, to have been benign. This phenomenon is true of imaging in general. Better images mean the detection of more potential problems, which can lead to expensive tests and treatments, some of them unnecessary.

After extensive Swedish studies showed little or no benefit from mammograms, some medical practitioners came out against early mammography: "The inescapable conclusion," write Jacquelyn Paykel and William Wolberg, "is that recommending screening in 40 to 49 year olds is a relatively costly step that is based on controversial data. . . . If the war against breast cancer is to be won, the focus of funding in this country must go beyond spending society's money on mammograms in order to provide better funding to explore new means of diagnosis, treatment and prevention."[4]

However, reducing the number of mammograms to cut costs must be balanced against the possibility that more cancers would go undetected. Michael Kinsley, founding editor of the online magazine *Slate*, observes: "Sure, the mere fact that a malignant tumor is caught by a mammogram doesn't mean that a woman's life has been saved: The tumor might have been discovered in time anyway, or something else might have killed her before the tumor could do its deadly work. But no one tries to deny that some tumors are caught and removed that would have been fatal and that some women are alive as a result."[5]

A Cost Crisis

The growing utility and sophistication of mammograms and other imaging technologies has brought on a funding crisis within the U.S. health-care system. In 2002 Medicare, the nation's largest government medical program, spent $6.5 billion on medical imaging. That represents one of every seven dollars in fees reimbursed by Medicare. Even that figure pales beside the estimated total expenditures for medical imaging. Management consulting firm Booz Allen Hamilton projects that spending on diagnostic imaging could grow by 28 percent in 2005 to reach a staggering $100 billion. An industry publication notes, "Ten years ago, medical imaging—including magnetic resonance imaging (MRIs), body scans and computed tomography imaging (CT scans)—wasn't even on the radar screen for most health insurers. In 2004, it's one of the highest-cost items in a health plan's medical budget, and also one of the fastest growing."[6]

Few patients pay the full expense of medical imaging directly out of pocket. Although most of the cost is borne by health insurers or the government, through programs such as Medicare, those costs are ultimately passed on to consumers and taxpayers. Faced with double-digit inflation in medical imaging, both government and the private sector have been exerting pressure on doctors and hospitals to limit imaging procedures. Early in 2005 Medicare drafted a report to Congress that proposed various measures to curb costs. One would be tracking physicians who overprescribe imaging for patients. Another measure would be to drive out wasteful operators by setting higher standards for those who perform medical imaging.

Similarly, private insurers are waging war on rising costs in imaging. Many are requiring physicians to get advance permission before sending a patient for imaging. Preauthorization, as this practice is called, results in as many as one in five requests being denied. Some insurers are encouraging patients to think twice about requesting expensive imaging services by tagging them with steep co-payments. Others are forcing participating physicians to undergo new certifications and abide by rules restricting the volume of imaging referrals they can make.

The Future of Imaging

How effective these steps might be remains uncertain. Many factors influence the frequency with which imaging procedures are prescribed and the resulting financial strain on America's health-care system. Manufacturers, who need to sell equipment to make profits, make continual improvements to the technology to find new market niches. Doctors, worried by the possibility of malpractice suits, feel pressured to offer the best available diagnosis. That can mean an expensive MRI instead of a routine X-ray for even a minor injury. "I don't want to say that all this new stuff is not worth the extra cost," Gary Claxton, vice president of the Kaiser Family Foundation, a research organization that studies health-care issues, told the *San Diego Union-Tribune*, "But it tends to cost more."[7]

The increasingly heavy costs of medical imaging will likely force health-care providers, the government, and insurers to restrict its use. A nation whose economy has on average grown by 3.3 percent annually since the mid-1990s and whose national debt has grown rapidly since 2000 cannot sustain double-digit inflation in health care. It may be that patients themselves, faced with crippling expenses for health insurance, will demand cost-cutting measures, which may include restrictions on expensive imaging procedures. Faced with higher co-pays, they may eschew some of these procedures. "In this era of cost-sharing, it appears, consumers are rationing their care on their own," observes the *Union Tribune* report.[8]

What consequences will follow the rationing of imaging procedures is hard to predict. Certainly medical costs will be reduced, but hopefully not at the expense of patient health. No physician would want to return to the pre-imaging era, where guesses were the only diagnostic tools available. To be sure, medical imaging is here to stay, so the challenge will be to use the procedures wisely so that rising expenses do not wind up reducing doctors' diagnostic tools.

Notes

1. Quoted in Pennsylvania State Universtity, "The Terrible Power of the Rays," 1993. www.xray.hmc.psu.edu.

2. Stanley J. Grossman and Landis K. Griffeth, "Usefulness of Positron Emission Tomography in Clinical Oncology," *Baylor University Medical Center Proceedings*, July 1999, p. 158.

3. National Institutes of Health, "Breast Cancer Screening for Women Ages 40–49," Consensus Development Conference Statement, January 21–23, 1997. http://concensus.nih.gov.

4. Jacqueline Paykel and William H. Wolberg, "Concerns About Recommending Routine Screening Mammograms for Women Age 40–49." www.wisc.edu.

5. Michael Kinsley, "What's the Down Side?" *Slate*, February 21, 2002. http:/slate.msn.com.

6. Quoted in AIShealth.com, "Controlling the Soaring Costs of Medical Imaging." www.aishealth.com.

7. Quoted in Leslie Berestein, "Insurance Ills Put Squeeze on Consumers: Sliding Benefits, Soaring Costs Swell Insurers' Profits," *San Diego Union-Tribune*, August 22, 2004. www.signonsandiego.com.

8. Berestein, "Insurance Ills Put Squeeze on Consumers."

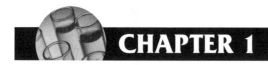

CHAPTER 1

The Early History of Medical Imaging

Before Imaging: An Ancient Greek View of Anatomy

By Galen

One of the most influential figures in medical history was the second-century Greek physician known as Galen. His views dominated Western medicine until at least the sixteenth century, when the Flemish anatomist Vesalius proved many of Galen's precepts wrong. For example, Galen taught that the heart has two chambers, when in fact it has four. However, as the following excerpt from his writings shows, Galen's understanding of anatomy was no worse and in many ways was better than to that of his peers.

A major topic of debate among ancient Greek physicians was whether blood flows through arteries, and if so how much. Galen, like his contemporaries, thought that blood was consumed as nourishment by the body. Therefore, they imagined that the flow of blood was one-way. Even so, he argues, correctly, that since the arteries connect with the veins, there must be an exchange of at least some blood between them. Physicians today know that all blood flows out from the heart through arteries and returns to it through veins. In the second section of this excerpt, he discusses the skeletal system. While his general inferences are sensible, he reveals that his knowledge of human anatomy comes from a few chance encounters with corpses. For the most part, he relied on animal bodies for actual studies, and this proved misleading. The problem for Galen and all other would-be physicians of the time was a long-standing taboo against human dissection. Galen advises others who would understand human anatomy to study the skeletons of apes. For many centuries, however, physicians ignored this advice and simply accepted his descriptions as dogma.

Galen was born about 130 A.D. in the town of Pergamum in Asia

Arthur J. Brock, *Greek Medicine: Being Extracts Illustrative of Medical Writers from Hippocrates to Galen*. New York: E.P. Dutton & Co., 1929.

Minor. He died around 200 A.D., leaving behind a wealth of philosophical and medical writings that earned him a reputation as the most famous physician in history after Hippocrates. Translator and editor Arthur J. Brock (1879–1947) was likewise a physician. In addition to renown for his translations, he is remembered for having treated poet Wilfred Owen for shell shock during World War I.

A lmost everybody agrees that, if certain important arteries are wounded in sufficient numbers, blood is evacuated through them. For this reason also even those people who, like Erasistratus [royal physician in Syria, c. 304–250 B.C.], do not allot any blood at all to the arteries, yet agree that they anastomose [connect] with the veins. In other words, although they think that Nature does everything *artistically*, and nothing in vain, yet they fail to realise that they are confessing that these anastomoses have been made for no purpose.

Yet by itself the fact that they were constructed in vain and are of no use to the animal would have been a small matter. But there is a fact more serious than this, and which one cannot any longer consider a small mistake on Nature's part; in other words, they admit logically that besides being no use, the arteries actually do a great deal of harm! Thus Erasistratus himself is at pains to point out to us the impossibility of any inflammation ever occurring without penetration (*paremptosis*) of blood from the veins into the arteries. Well then, if it is impossible for inflammation to occur otherwise, living beings would no longer be troubled by pleurisy, nor phrenitis, nor peripneumonia, if these anastomoses [junctures between veins and arteries] were done away with! Nay, there would be no ophthalmia nor quinsy nor angina if these did not exist. And of course there would be no inflammation either of the liver, the stomach, the spleen, or anything else. What more? Most of the worst diseases would no longer occur were there none of these anastomoses, created by the providence of Nature not to perform any useful function for the animal, but destined to be merely organs of deadly disease! Nor, of course, would inflammation follow wounds if the anastomoses were not there, nor would fever supervene upon plethora, nor would inflammation occur in the liver, the alimentary canal, the heart, or in any of the other organs where it most quickly causes death!

Roles of Blood Vessels

Now I have already discussed not merely once or twice, but many times and in many ways, the hypothesis of Erasistratus about the arteries, to show how far this contradicts and is opposed to an obvious fact, and I think it superfluous to go into the matter here. For Nature has not created the anastomoses of arteries with veins idly or at random, but in order that the benefit derived from respiration and pulsation may be distributed, not only to the heart and arteries, but also to the veins. I have written elsewhere about the amount of benefit they thus receive; for our present purposes it is enough to know the facts.

And, further, the fact lately mentioned, that all parts of the body do not require the same nourishment, itself shows the value of vessels of different origin. If there was only one kind of vessel—the blood-vessel—all parts of the body would have similar nourishment. Now this is quite unreasonable—in fact it is absolutely absurd—that the same blood should be used as nourishment of, let us say, both liver and lungs, that is the heaviest and densest of the viscera as against the lightest and most spongy. This is why Nature has very properly made in living bodies not arteries only, but veins as well. And hence the liver is nourished by veins alone, and by the very finest and most permeable of these, and the lung by arteries; indeed the veins of the lung, in so far as they provide nourishment, also resemble arteries. We must admire therefore the forethought of Nature in providing vessels of two kinds, and in anastomosing their adjacent ends with each other—and even before that, in doing the same thing with the cavities of the heart. . . .

The fossæ [cavities] which appear on the septum in the middle of the heart exist to subserve the communication of which I speak. For in any case it would be better for the arteries to receive the blood which has been previously elaborated in the veins; then the veins would be in the same position with respect to the arteries as the stomach is with respect to the veins. For logically it is not impossible that the psychic pneuma is a kind of exhalation of useful blood. This also has been discussed at greater length elsewhere. Enough for our present purpose to mention the value of the arteries containing clear, thin blood which is destined at least to nourish the psychic pneuma.

All these, then, are strong proofs of how well Nature has done to provide these two kinds of vessels. And, furthermore, there is

the fact that the arteries need a certain strength—in fact, a coat—
as they have to be in constant motion. Now this coat cannot be
strong and thin at the same time, while, if it becomes thick, many
parts of the body would not be suitably nourished.

Nature, then, has very properly made all these arrangements
throughout the body, and first of all in the heart itself, where it has
devised a communication of veins with arteries by means of these
narrow openings (*stomata*). For the same reason the vein [vena
cava] opening into the heart is greater than that proceeding from
it [pulmonary artery], although the latter vein receives the blood
poured into it by virtue of the heart's heat; since a great deal of
blood passes through the intervening septum and its fossæ into the
left ventricle, it is natural that the vein proceeding to the lungs
should be smaller than that which brings blood into the heart. And
similarly also the artery [pulmonary vein] which brings the
pneuma from the lung to the heart is itself much smaller than the
great artery [aorta] from which all the arteries throughout the body
arise, since the great artery receives some blood from the right
ventricle, and is destined to become the source of all the arteries
of the organism. . . .

The Skeletal System

What tent-poles are to tents, and walls to houses, so to animals is
their bony structure; the other parts adapt themselves to this, and
change with it. Thus, if an animal's cranium is round, its brain
must be the same; or, again, if it is oblong, then the animal's brain
must also be oblong. If the jaws are small, and the face as a whole
roundish, the muscles of these parts will also necessarily be small;
and similarly, if the jaws are prominent, the animal's face as a
whole will be long, as also the facial muscles. Consequently also
the monkey (*pithēcus*) is of all animals the likest to man in its viscera, muscles, arteries, veins, and nerves (*neura*), because it is so
also in the form of its bones. From the nature of these it walks on
two legs, uses its front limbs as hands, has the flattest breast-bone
of all quadrupeds, collar-bones like those of a man, a round face
and a short neck. And these being similar, the muscles cannot be
different; for they are extended on the outside of the bones in such
a manner that they resemble them in size and form. To the muscles, again, correspond the arteries, veins, and nerves; so these,
being similar, must correspond to the bones.

The Importance of Bones

First of all, then, I would ask you to make yourself well acquainted with the human bones, and not to look on this as a matter of secondary importance. Nor must you merely read the subject up in one of these books which are called by some "Osteology," by others "The Skeleton," and by others simply "On Bones," as is my own book; which, by the way, I am certain is better than any previously written, both as regards the exactitude of its matter and the brevity and clearness of its explanations. Make it your earnest business, then, not only to learn exactly from the book the appearance of each of the bones, but to become yourself by the use of your own eyes an eager first-hand observer of human osteology.

At Alexandria this is very easy, since the physicians in that country accompany the instruction they give to their students with opportunities for personal inspection (*autopsia*). Hence you must try to get to Alexandria for this reason alone, if for no other. But if you cannot manage this, still it is not impossible to obtain a view of human bones. Personally I have very often had a chance to do this where tombs or monuments have become broken up. On one occasion a river, having risen to the level of a grave which had been carelessly constructed a few months previously, easily disintegrated this; then by the force of its current it swept right over the dead man's body, of which the flesh had already putrefied, while the bones were still closely attached to one another. This it carried away down-stream for the distance of a league, till, coming to a lake-like stretch with sloping banks, it here deposited the corpse. And here the latter lay ready for inspection, just as though prepared by a doctor for his pupil's lesson.

Once also I examined the skeleton of a robber, lying on a mountain-side a short distance from the road. This man had been killed by some traveller whom he had attacked, but who had been too quick for him. None of the inhabitants of the district would bury him; but in their detestation of him they were delighted when his body was eaten by birds of prey; the latter, in fact, devoured the flesh in two days and left the skeleton ready, as it were, for anyone who cared to enjoy an anatomical demonstration.

Apes Will Do

As regards yourself, then, even if you do not have the luck to see anything like this, still you can dissect an ape, and learn each of the bones from it, by carefully removing the flesh. For this purpose you must choose the apes which most resemble man. Such are those in whom the jaws are not prominent nor the canine teeth large. In such apes you will also find the other parts as in man, whence they walk and run on two legs. Those of them, again, that are like the dog-headed baboon (*cynocephalæ*) have longer muzzles and large canine teeth; they have difficulty in standing upright on two legs, let alone walking about or running.

But even those apes most like human beings fall somewhat short of the absolutely erect posture. In them the head of the femur is adjusted somewhat obliquely to the hip-socket, and certain of the muscles which run down to the tibia come far forward; both of these factors impair or prevent assumption of the erect posture, as also do their feet, for in these the heels are somewhat narrow and the toes widely separated from each other. These, however, are small matters, and so the ape comes very near being able to stand erect.

Those monkeys which resemble the dog-faced baboons and have a marked divergence from the human type show also as clear difference in their bones. Choose, therefore, among the monkeys the most men-like (*anthropoid*), and learn accurately on them the nature of the bones, comparing them with my writings. You will also have to accustom yourself without delay to their names, as these will also be useful in learning the anatomy of other parts.

Thus if you should also later meet with a human skeleton, you would easily recognise and remember everything. If, on the other hand, you content yourself with reading only, without familiarising yourself beforehand with the sight of the ape's bones, you will neither recognise accurately a human skeleton if you suddenly see one, nor will you be able to remember it; for in order to keep in mind sensible facts, constant familiarity is needed. This is the reason why also among men we quickly recognise those with whom we have often had to do, whereas if we see a person only once or twice and meet him again after any length of time, we pass him by, failing entirely to recognise him or even to remember our previous meeting. Consequently also the far-famed "fortuitous anatomy" to which some physicians pay honour is not an adequate way of learning the nature of the parts visible. We must have plenty of leisure to inspect each of the parts first, so that, when suddenly seen, it may be recognised. And this should be done preferably with actual human beings, and, if not with them, then with animals like them.

Listening to the Body: A History of the Early Stethoscope

By D.M. Cammann

The most significant diagnostic instrument prior to the advent of medical imaging was the stethoscope, which allowed doctors to hear what was going on inside their patients' chests. In the following selection a nineteenth-century physician relates a history of the stethoscope. The text comes from an address by D.M. Cammann, who contributed his own improvement to the device. His address was originally published in the *New York Medical Journal* in 1886.

Acknowledging that others had previously paved the way, Cammann begins by describing the pioneering work of French physician Rene Laennec, who is widely credited with constructing the first crude stethoscope around 1816. Laennec's first attempt involved rolling up sheets of paper into a listening tube. Pierre Piorry followed up this prototype with a stiff, wood-and-ivory tube. In 1843, Cammann writes, a Dr. Williams created trumpet-shaped stethoscopes. Cammann credits a French physician with creating the binaural (for two ears) stethoscope sometime before 1850. He also refers to Dr. George P. Cammann (1804–1863), the man most historians credit with creating the prototype of the modern flexible stethoscope. The Cammann stethoscope, created around 1852, had ivory earpieces connected to flexible tubes that met in a hollow ball just above the chestpiece. George Cammann made his instrument freely available to the medical profession without patent, and its use quickly spread. The author describes his own improvement to the original model: a vacuum bulb that makes the chestpiece adhere to the chest.

D.M. Cammann, "An Historic Sketch of the Stethoscope," *New York Medical Journal*, April 24, 1996.

D.M. Cammann was a physician in New York. His precise relationship to George Cammann is unknown.

I will not consider whether the idea of the stethoscope originated with Hippocrates, Bayle, Hook, or [Rene] Laennec.
Laennec made the idea practically useful. His first instrument
was a cylinder of paper compactly rolled and kept in shape by
paste. The longitudinal aperture, always left in the center of the
paper thus rolled, led accidentally, in his hands, to its discovery.
The stethoscope that he subsequently adopted was a cylinder of
wood, an inch and a half in diameter and a foot long, perforated
longitudinally by a bore three lines wide and hollowed out into a
funnel shape at one end to the depth of an inch and a half.

[Pierre] Piorry introduced a more slender instrument with ivory
cap, and later this was altered and made of wood only. Instruments
with a trumpet-shaped end were devised by Dr. Williams about
1843. Since then the modifications of the monaural stethoscope
have been numerous and more than thirty may be found scattered
through the files of medical journals. Some have been hollow and
others solid. They have been made of wood, metal, vulcanite,
papier-mache, and other materials, either alone or in combination.
Among others may be mentioned the stethoscopes of Walshe,
Quain, Loomis, Cammann, and Clark. Previous to 1850, M. Landouzy, of Paris, constructed a binaural instrument having a number of gum-elastic tubes by which several persons could listen at
once. This required three hands for its application and was not
found of any practical use. Many years before this, Dr. Williams,
of London, was accustomed to a stethoscope made of two metal
tubes attached to the bell of an ordinary stethoscope with flat ear-
pieces. This conveyed sounds with exaggerated intensity, but was
inflexible and awkward of application. The double stethoscope of
Dr. [Arthur] Leared, shown at the International Exhibition of
1851, was a great improvement. It consisted of two gutta-percha
tubes attached to the ear-pieces. These tubes, being drawn apart
and applied to the ears, were kept in place by their own elasticity.

Cammann's Unpatented Stethoscope

In 1851, Dr. Marsh, of Cincinnatti, patented a double stethoscope.
This had a membrane stretching over its objective end, and two

gum-elastic tubes leading from the chest-piece to the ears. In this instrument the ear-pieces were inconvenient; it required two hands for its application, and the sounds conveyed were muffled and confused. These circumstances rendered it of little value. Dr. [George] Cammann was familiar with these two instruments, Landouzy's and Marsh's, and it was chiefly the fact that Marsh's was patented which induced Dr. Cammann to devise a better one and give it freely to the profession. His binaural stethoscope, therefore, was not a new invention, but was, and is now, the best instrument of the kind devised. It was only after much labor and considerable expense that a satisfactory result was attained. The instrument was perfected in 1852, and described in the "New York Medical Times" of January, 1855. It is light, durable, easily carried, and a good conductor of sound. The ear-pieces are the best that have been devised, but room for improvement in this respect still remains. The attachment of a rim of soft rubber to the chest-piece, as debased by Dr. Snelling, is of advantage in applying it more closely to the inequalities of the chest. In most of the instruments now made the rubber band which serves to draw the two tubes together is replaced by a spring. In the latest improvement the spring is placed in the screw which binds the tubes together.

Great care is required in the construction of the stethoscope, and many defective ones are sold. The knobs on the ear-pieces must neither be too large nor too small; if too small, they cause pain by their pressure; if too large, they allow external sounds to enter the ear. The tubes must be curved so that they enter the ear in the direction of the meatus. The flexible tubes must not be too stiff nor too long, and their movements must be noiseless.

Many Variations

A considerable variety of flexible stethoscopes is now [1886] in use. They may be generally described as consisting of a chest-piece, long flexible rubber tubes, and round ear-pieces. The ear-pieces are held in place wither by being firmly pressed into the meatus, or by a spring passing over the head or under the chin. A flexible stethoscope is described by Mr. Brown in the "Lancet," March 3, 1877, in which the ear-pieces are oval. When placed in the ear with the long diameter vertical, they are said to remain readily in position. The differential stethoscope of Scott Alison is similar in mechanism to Cammann's, but had two chest-pieces—

one for each ear, enabling the sounds from different regions of the chest to be conveyed to the ears at the same time. The value of this stethoscope has been a matter of considerable controversy. It is claimed that it is capable of offering aid in diagnosis in two ways:

(1) By the consecutive observation of the sounds of two regions of the chest by the different ears, and (2) by their simultaneous observation. We can listen over different parts of the chest with either ear by removing one or the other chest-piece, and thus can compare the sounds heard over different regions with great rapidity, and detect slight differences which might escape us in a prolonged examination. If we listen at two points simultaneously, and sound of the same quality but of different intensity is heard at each point, the weaker is eclipsed or nullified, and thus, by the eclipsing of a weaker impression through one ear by a stronger impression through the other, differences may be recognized which might otherwise escape detection. When hearing is impaired in one ear, this stethoscope can not be used satisfactorily.

Making Use of Water

The hydrophone is another instrument devised by Alison. It consists of an India-rubber bag about the size of a large watch and filled with water. Another inventor had previously constructed a wooden instrument filled with water, but it was not practically useful. Alison found that when water was interposed between two conducting media, sound was conveyed to the ear with greater intensity. The hydrophone may be employed as an instrument by itself or in aid of the stethoscope. The increase of sound varies much with the material through which it is conducted. With firm, non-flexible, or solid stethoscopes, the hydrophone acts as a damper and diminishes sound. The more a stethoscope becomes a mere air instrument and departs from the character of a solid conducting medium, the more water adds to its acoustic value. This may explain why such opposite results have been obtained in the use of the hydrophone by different observers.

Some years ago the idea of a stethoscope containing an air-chamber in the chest-piece was suggested by Dr. Learning. In 1884 ("Diseases of the Heart," by Constantin Paul, William Wood & Co., 1884) Dr. Constantin Paul devised a stethoscope with two flexible tubes leading to the ears, and a hollow chamber in the chest-piece, connected with a rubber bulb by a long flexible tube.

If the air in the hollow chamber is exhausted, the instrument is held firmly against the chest.

Adding a Suction Cup

My modification of Cammann's stethoscope ("New York Medical Journal," January 3, 1885) can be screwed on in place of the usual chest-piece.

In the pectoral end is an air-chamber which is completely closed by pressure against the chest, the inner and outer rims of the chamber being on the same level. Connected with this chamber by a small tubular opening is a rubber bulb through which the sound conducting tube passes. By pressure upon this bulb when the instrument is held in position, the air is exhausted in the hollow chamber, and the stethoscope is held firmly to the chest-wall. It requires some practice to use this modification successfully. The bulb should be strongly compressed, and then firm and even pressure made against the chest-wall, when the pressure upon the bulb should be at once relaxed. If this be done, the instrument is held in place during the examination, or at least for a considerable time.

I have used this instrument for more than a year, and am confirmed in my opinion of its value. By its use the closest possible contact is obtained with the parts under examination. Sound, in passing to the ear, is conveyed through two hollow chambers— one in the chest-piece, and the rubber bulb—both of which act as resonators and increase its intensity. Not only is the intensity of the sounds increased, but their true quality is better appreciated. Another advantage is that the two hands of the auscultator [person listening to the chest] are left free to practice the method of auscultatory percussion—a method which has not yet received the attention it deserves, and which, it is to be hoped, will come into more general use.

The Discovery of X-Rays

By Neil Sclater

Many discoveries in science occur not in pursuit of some particular technology, but simply to satisfy the curiosity of scientists about how nature works. Often, this so-called basic research brings totally unforeseen benefits in another field. The following selection begins with one of the most famous instances of scientific serendipity: the discovery of X-rays, which led to the first medical imaging tool.

Technology writer Neil Sclater describes how in 1895 German scientist Wilhelm Röntgen followed up the experiments of others on cathode rays (electron beams). These were generated in vacuum tubes by shooting a powerful electric current from one node to another. In particular, Röntgen was following in the footsteps of British physicist William Crookes, who very nearly discovered X-rays himself. However, it fell to Röntgen to achieve the unexpected breakthrough. While experimenting in a darkened room with an electric tube, he noticed that it caused a chemically treated paper to glow. When he placed his hand between the tube and the paper, he discovered that an image of the flesh and bones of his hand formed on the paper. After further investigation, Röntgen was able to demonstrate how X-rays could be used to reveal the body's internal anatomy. Since then, Sclater relates, X-ray technology has undergone considerable refinement, permitting clear images at much lower dosages. Neil Sclater is the author of six books and many articles on engineering subjects.

Neil Sclater, "X-Rays and Their Discoverer," *Electronics Now*, vol. 66, November 1995, pp. 29–30. Reproduced by permission.

"**H**unch your shoulders forward, take a deep breath—and don't breathe or move! Ready?" This is what you hear from your physician or a technician before the buzz and click that tells you invisible rays have passed through your body and impinged on photographic film. Having X-ray pictures taken at a physician's or dentist's office is the way most people are deliberately exposed to this high-frequency radiation—and then for only a fraction of a second.

The large X-ray negative tells the physician a lot about your heart, lungs and other internal organs. No needles, tongue depressors, chest thumping, or other invasive procedures. And it tells a lot about the properties of X-rays—their ability to penetrate cloth, paper and flesh to reveal, in shadowy outline, the presence of disease, the location of bone fractures or the presence of foreign bodies.

But there is nothing new here, you say, you knew all this. Most of us take the X-ray exam for granted, and could not visualize modern medicine without it. So why raise the subject at this time? The answer is that X-rays were first discovered, quite by accident, one hundred years ago this month [November 1995].

What is more, the role for X-rays is still expanding from its original—and perhaps still most important one—in medical diagnostics. However, X-rays are also used to treat cancers, analyze materials, detect contraband, inspect the quality of welds, and even reveal more about the universe. Although still in the experimental stage, X-ray lithography holds promise for sub-micrometer, high-density integrated circuit fabrication. And, don't forget the X-ray television and X-ray lasers.

Building on the Work of Others

On November 8, 1895, physics professor Wilhelm Konrad Röntgen (often Anglicized to Roentgen) (1845–1923), was working in his laboratory at the Physical Institute at the University of Wurzburg, Germany, trying to duplicate and understand the results of experiments done by others in the emerging field of electrical conduction through a vacuum or gas.

Professor Röntgen knew what the others had accomplished, and he had all of the apparatus needed to permit him to duplicate their findings. Fortunately for science, medicine, and mankind, he was a trained scientist who quickly recognized the value of his discovery and lost no time in trumpeting it to the world. But before saying more about how Dr. Röntgen discovered X-rays, the work of the other scientists, principally English and German, should be put in perspective so you can appreciate the fortuitous circumstances surrounding his discovery.

Perhaps you recall reading about Heinrich Geissler (1814–1891), a German instrument maker, master glass blower, and physicist from the article "Seeing the Unseen" in the October 1995 *Electronics Now*. In the 1850s Geissler invented a gas-filled, light-emitting tube that produced a controlled, continuous source of bright light. He accomplished what he set out to do—develop a source of continuous light for spectroscopy, but later it was found that his tube could be pulsed. It became the ancestor of the modern flashlamp.

Geissler also contributed to the development of the modern vacuum pump, necessary equipment for evacuating closed tubes for all experiments in electron conduction through vacuum and gas tubes. About that same time, the English physicist Michael Faraday (1791–1867), best known for his pioneering work in electromagnetic induction and the discoverer of the basic principles of the electric motor, was also investigating electricity in gas-filled tubes.

Others active in the field at the time were the German physicists Johann Wilhelm Hittorf and Julius Plucker. Hittorf named the mysterious flow of electricity in tube "cathode rays," but we now know that they were really streams of electrons. During the next 20 years Plucker, Hittorf, and others in Germany revealed most of the important characteristics of ionized gas and cathode rays.

To carry out their experiments, those scientists needed power supplies. Most started off by wiring large batteries in series, and some even tried friction machines. Eventually they turned to the battery-powered induction coil. It was compact, portable, and easily controlled by a switch in the primary circuit. During the 1850s, another German instrument maker, Heinrich Ruhmkorff, improved the coil by separating the primary and secondary coils with a glass bobbin. Later interrupters, formed by moving wires in and out of a mercury pool, were installed for switching the primary windings.

In 1875 the English physicist, Sir William Crookes (1832–1919) improved on the Geissler tube, and in 1879 he demonstrated peculiar glow phenomena by passing current through a cathode tube that contained traces of gas. Crookes found that if the air pressure in the tube is reduced by a vacuum pump to about 1 centimeter of mercury, a thin bright streamer can be seen between the anode and cathode of the tube. Its color depends on the gas in the tube.

As the pressure is lowered further, the streamer is replaced by a bright column of light filling the whole space between the electrodes. This was the stage reached in Geissler tube and in modern neon and argon lamps. If the pressure is reduced further to about 1 millimeter of mercury, the positive space shrinks and dark spaces appear.

Finally the column disappears entirely, and, the pressure at about 0.001 millimeter of mercury, the walls of the tube glow with a greenish light (fluorescence). Crookes did not know it then, but this stage must be reached to cause X-ray radiation. The phenomena produced also depends on the size of the tube and the impressed voltage. However, Crookes discovered that the cathode rays could cast a shadow on fluorescent material at the end of the tube.

Crookes' demonstrations inspired other scientists to experiment with cathode rays passing through glass tubes with partial vacuums, gas, and combinations of these. The flow of electricity in the Crookes tubes was initiated by an induction coil. . . . The electrons that formed the current originated at the cathode and passed through the partial vacuum to the anode.

Missed Opportunity

Ironically, photographic plates that Crookes kept in his laboratory were mysteriously fogged and ruined, although they were in protective containers, but he never knew why. Thus, he missed his opportunity to discover X-rays. The effects he produced could not be explained with the physics of the day—much as science today cannot explain the phenomena known as ball lightning.

Now back to Professor Röntgen. On that fateful day in 1895, he set out to study discharge from a Crookes tube so he could explain the phenomena. His apparatus was the same as that used by Crookes, and it included a Ruhmkorff coil. Because the Crookes tube glowed slightly when the current flowed, Röntgen darkened the room to see the glow better. He also covered the end of the tube with black cardboard to block the cathode rays.

However, much to his annoyance he noticed a fluorescent glow from a sheet of paper coated with a barium salt across the room. He looked around for the cause of the fluorescence and saw only that the Crookes tube was operating. But the end of the tube was still covered. He shut off the power and saw that the glow of the paper faded, and the room was dark again.

After turning the tube back on the greenish glow reappeared. He put a book in front of the tube and the paper still glowed. Then he replaced the book with a block of wood and even used rubber as a shield, but the strange radiation passed right through. He then put a box of laboratory weights in front of the tube and found that dark silhouettes of the weights showed up on the paper screen.

Finally, he placed his hand between the tube and distant coated paper and was astonished to see the faint outline of the flesh of his hand and the dark outline of the bones. Next, he made the first intentional X-ray photograph by asking his wife to put her hand between the tube and a photographic plate. That's when he knew he was on to something.

His observations drove Dr. Röntgen to carry out more experiments to confirm that what he saw actually happened and could be reproduced. The Crookes tube was indeed the source of the mysterious invisible rays. Because, at the time, he could not explain them, he called them X-rays. At the end of December in 1895 Professor Röntgen submitted his first paper on the mysterious rays.

In January of 1896 Professor Röntgen gave the first public demonstration of X-rays. Soon scientists in laboratories around the world had duplicated his results. More than a thousand scientific articles were published on X-rays within a year of their discovery!

Winner of a Nobel Prize

Although Professor Röntgen never became wealthy as a result of his discovery, he did gain the recognition of the world's scientific community. In 1901, Dr. Röntgen became the first physicist to receive a Nobel prize. However, in 1903 a French scientist, Antoine Becquerel, also received a Nobel prize for the discovery of natural radiation. Today this term means radioactivity and it includes alpha, beta, and gamma rays. Gamma rays are more energetic than X-rays and they generally have shorter wavelengths and higher frequencies. Otherwise, they have the same general characteristics. . . .

Primitive Versus Modern Equipment

The Crookes tube was pretty simple. It was, in effect, a vacuum tube diode without a plate. Electrons emitted from the cathode are accelerated by the charge on the anode, which in his tube was only a wire. Thus, some of the radiation bypasses the small anode and exits through the end of the glass tube. If the voltage on the anode is high enough, X-rays will be produced by the collision of electrons with the glass of the tube. . . .

When high-speed electrons strike a massive target such as one made of lead or tungsten, X-rays are generated. This X-ray tube contains a heated cathode that emits electrons as in most vacuum tubes and the anode target, typically made of tungsten embedded in a water-cooled copper block. The tungsten resists the destructive effects of heat caused by the energetic electron bombardment. The anode surface is beveled to deflect the X-rays, and the gap between the cathode and the anode is only a few inches.

The heated cathode emits electrons, and the anode has a positive voltage. It is essentially a vacuum-tube diode. A high-voltage power supply accelerates the electrons which strike the anode at an angle of about 45°. As a consequence, X-rays are scattered in all directions, but most focused into a cone whose axis is at right angles to the centerline of the tube.

Conventional X-ray radiograms view the body from only one angle. The rays are absorbed (shadowed) by dense objects like bones, artificial joints, and metal foreign objects. However, the softer tissues—muscles, organs, and skin are more easily penetrated. X-ray films or radiograms represent the amount of X-ray penetration with different gray (intensity) levels.

Over the past 20 years, the introduction of image-intensifier technology in X-ray machines has permitted a significant reduction in the duration and intensity of the X-ray to which the patient are exposed without sacrificing picture sharpness and quality.

Some new X-ray systems include electronics that can scan and digitize the image and send signals to a closed circuit television set for such functions as real-time inspection of welds without endangering the operator of the inspection equipment.

Some X-ray systems include electronics that can scan the image and, by means of Xerography, produce an instant picture on paper. This saves the time lost and expense of manually developing a photographic film. These systems are not likely to replace conventional X-ray equipment because there is a tradeoff in detail. However, they can cut the cost of routine physical exams, and they can be life-savers in situations where surgeons are treating severe trauma victims. No time is lost waiting for a negative to be developed.

One of the most innovative X-ray systems developed within the past 25 years [prior to 1995] is computer-aided tomography, now generally called computed tomography (CT). This system, a marriage between the X-ray machine and a computer, converts signals generated by X-rays into video images of a cross section of a patient.

The Origins of Magnetic Resonance Imaging

By The Economist

Magnetic resonance imaging (MRI) has taken its place alongside
X-rays and ultrasound as one of the most important medical imaging
technologies. For obtaining detailed images of soft tissues, such as
the brain, it is unsurpassed. MRI has now been in use for several
decades. Yet, as the following selection from *The Economist* news
magazine shows, a controversy over who should get credit for its invention continues to rage. Paul Lauterbur and Peter Mansfield shared
a 2003 Nobel Prize for discoveries leading to the invention of MRI.
Far from settling the question, however, this award only intensified
the dispute, according to the magazine. Physician Raymond Damadian, who considers himself the true inventor of the technology, responded to the award granting with full-page newspaper advertisements demanding the Nobel committee reconsider its decision. The
committee declined to do so, and the controversy persists. Damadian's
contributions have not gone unrecognized, however. In 1988 President Ronald Reagan awarded him the National Medal of Technology,
and in 2001 the Lemelson-MIT Program at the Massachusetts Institute of Technology gave him a lifetime achievement prize.

The Economist, founded in 1843 by a Scottish manufacturer to
promote free trade, is now published throughout the world. It covers
subjects that affect business and the economy.

The Economist, "MRI's Inside Story," vol. 369, December 6, 2003, p. 26. Copyright © 2003 by
The Economist Newspaper Ltd., www.economist.com. All rights reserved. Reproduced by permission.

"You know, what these people do is really very clever. They put little spies into the molecules and send radio signals to them, and they have to radio back what they are seeing." That is how the physicist Niels Bohr is said to have described the principles behind magnetic-resonance imaging (MRI). Since its emergence in the 1970s, MRI has become a vital tool for diagnosing brain tumours and other diseases of the central nervous system, and for spotting soft-tissue injuries in muscles and ligaments. Functional MRI, a newer and even cleverer technology, provides real-time information on brain activity, which is particularly useful in guiding neurosurgeons. Unlike X-rays, magnetic resonance is completely harmless and provides far more detailed images of soft tissues. About 22,000 MRI machines around the world were used in 60 [million] examinations last year [2002].

In October [2003], Paul Lauterbur, the director of the Biomedical Imaging Centre at the University of Illinois in Urbana-Champaign, and Sir Peter Mansfield, a physicist at the University of Nottingham in Britain, received the Nobel prize in medicine for making discoveries that "led to the development of modern magnetic-resonance imaging". Many in the field believe the award of a prize for the invention of MRI has been long overdue. But the decision has re-ignited a long-standing controversy surrounding one man—Raymond Damadian—who regards himself as the true inventor of MRI, and claims that this year's winners made technological improvements based on his discovery. Others, however, describe Dr Damadian as a doctor with a big ego who had a good idea, but contributed little to its ultimate technical realisation. So who is right?

MRI has a complex history, even without the hoopla over Dr Damadian. It was made possible by contributions from numerous visionary scientists—including a handful of Nobel prize winners—over a period of more than 50 years, incorporating bits and pieces from many different disciplines, such as chemistry, mathematics, engineering, computer science, medicine and, of course, physics.

A Nobel Prize for NMR

Felix Bloch of Stanford and Edward Purcell of Harvard shared the Nobel prize in 1952 for developing a way to measure the phenomenon that underpins MRI: nuclear magnetic resonance (NMR). The nuclei of atoms behave like tiny, spinning bar magnets. When placed in a strong, static magnetic field, nuclei tend to align with it, much like compass needles. When zapped with pulse of radio waves, the nuclei absorb energy, become "excited" and change direction. The time it takes them to "relax" and return to their original state can be measured. Because many different atomic nuclei resonate at a characteristic radio frequency in a given magnetic field, NMR spectroscopy is now widely used to determine the molecular make-up of chemical compounds.

In the late 1960s, Dr Damadian, at the time a physician at State University of New York's medical centre in Brooklyn, was among the first to contemplate using NMR to scan the human body for disease. Following an obscure theory devised by Gilbert Ling, a physiologist, Dr Damadian believed he would be able to distinguish cancerous from healthy tissues on the basis of the cells' water structure. Most scientists consider Dr Ling's ideas wacky at best. Undeterred, Dr Damadian experimented by analysing excised tumours of rats using machines at NMR Specialties, a now-defunct company based in New Kensington, Pennsylvania. He found that the hydrogen nuclei of water in cancerous and healthy tissues showed pronounced differences in relaxation times, an observation he published in the journal *Science* in 1971.

Around the same time, Dr Lauterbur, then president of NMR Specialties, spent some time observing another research team that had come to the company to repeat Dr Damadian's experiments. One momentous night, while eating at a local diner with a colleague, Dr Lauterbur had the idea that is now at the core of how MRI scanners operate: to superimpose small variations, or gradients, in the uniform magnetic field normally used in NMR spectroscopy. Changing the field strength affects the resonance frequency of nuclei in direct proportion, and can thus be used to collect spatial information. The intensity of the resonance signal at a particular frequency then indicates the quantity of a given kind of nucleus in a particular location. (Most MRI scanners are tuned to detect hydrogen nuclei, which are abundant in the body's tissues in the form of water.)

It was a groundbreaking insight, says Michael Moseley, president of the International Society for Magnetic Resonance in Medicine. At the time, many scientists thought creating a diagnostic imaging device based on NMR seemed far-fetched, if not ludicrous. Dr Moseley admits to being one of the sceptics initially. Most NMR machines, then chemists' tools, were made up of hollow magnets that could hold a sample the size of a pen. They also required a stringently uniform magnetic field that enabled chemists to measure the small differences in magnetic fields within molecules, essential to determining a specimen's molecular make-up. Such systems were, however, useless for detecting spatial information.

A Feud over Credit

In 1973, Dr Lauterbur published his idea in *Nature* along with the first MR images, of two tiny tubes filled with water. But his paper did not cite Dr Damadian's *Science* paper, even though Dr Lauterbur made a direct reference to it in a notebook entry made the day after his own discovery. When Dr Damadian found out that he had not been credited, he was livid. "One of the reasons for the bitter antagonism between the two people was that Lauterbur never referenced Damadian," recalls Lawrence Minkoff, a former student and employee of Dr Damadian.

Not long after Dr Lauterbur's paper appeared in *Nature*, he began to promote the possibilities of MRI or "zeugmatography" as he called it, and fellow researchers took note. The mid-1970s saw a flurry of activity in the area. Against a backdrop of scepticism, teams at a handful of universities in America and Britain raced to publish images of ever increasing complexity. Soon the covers and pages of esteemed scientific journals featured images of such objects as a mouse, a finger, a lemon, a wrist and, finally, a human head. The eventual goal: to build a whole-body scanner.

Extravagant Claim

Dr Damadian was determined to win that race. In the early 1970s, he had devised his own method of scanning the human body point by point, originally intended to produce data rather than pictures. Nonetheless, Field Focusing Nuclear Magnetic Resonance (FONAR) was the method used when he captured headlines in 1977, publishing the first image of a chest cavity of a live man. Initially, he had volunteered his own body for the job—without success. His associates told him he was too fat, recalls Dr Damadian. Indeed, "Indomitable", which is what he called his machine, preferred Dr Minkoff's skinny torso. On July 3rd, 1977, after four hours and 45 minutes of collecting data from 106 points, a picture was created.

In characteristic fashion, Dr Damadian sent out a press release claiming he had created "a new technique for the non-surgical detection of cancer anywhere in the human body." At that point, however, the machine had not been tested on cancer patients. When experts questioned Dr Damadian's assertion, he was forced to back down. In fact, that first full-body scanner, now on view at the National Inventors Hall of Fame in Akron, Ohio, on loan from the Smithsonian National Museum of American History, was an incredibly crude machine. A few years later, even Dr Damadian himself abandoned its underlying technology.

Meanwhile, Sir Peter Mansfield, who had also suggested gradients as a way to spatially localise NMR signals in a paper published in 1973, further contributed to the development of MRI by devising a scheme to acquire MR signals and construct images rapidly. When he presented his ideas at a symposium in 1977, he recalls facing a silent audience. Sir Peter wasn't entirely surprised, since his method could theoretically speed up the process of producing images from an hour to a fraction of a second. Because of the hardware requirements, it took more than a decade to implement his "echo-planar" imaging technique, but it is now commonly used to watch the brain at work in functional MRI.

Other researchers made their mark on the field, such as Richard Ernst, a Swiss scientist. Originally, Dr Lauterbur collected spatial information by rotating the gradient around an object. Dr Ernst suggested positioning gradients to form a rectangular grid, to simplify the process of creating two-dimensional images. In 1980, two British teams—one from Aberdeen University, the other a collaboration between EMI and Hammersmith Hospital—developed ways to optimise the contrast of images using differences in relaxation times. The Aberdeen group also came up with a practical implementation of Dr Ernst's technique, known as "spin warp" imaging, the method most commonly used for MRI today. In 1991, Dr Ernst was rewarded with a Nobel prize for chemistry.

Corporations Get Involved

With the development of more sophisticated whole-body MRI prototypes in 1980, interest in the new technology mounted. Corporations began to grasp that MRI (the word "nuclear" had been dropped for marketing reasons by this time) might become a useful adjunct to computer tomography (CT) scans, which create detailed images by combining multiple X-ray images. Philips, Johnson & Johnson, General Electric and other corporate heavyweights decided to pour millions into the promising technology.

As many researchers moved into the commercial sector, Dr Damadian did not sit idle. In 1978, he founded FONAR, based in Melville, New York. The small company struggled against its mighty competitors. But Dr Damadian's patents, the first one granted for an "apparatus and method for detecting cancer in tissue" in 1974, proved extremely useful. In 1997, after a lengthy legal fight that ended up in the Supreme Court of the United States, General Electric was ordered to pay FONAR nearly $130 [million] for patent infringement. Cases with other companies were settled for undisclosed sums.

Dr Damadian achieved success in court, and received America's National Medal of Technology together with Paul Lauterbur in 1988. (In September this year [2003], he won an Innovation Award in bioscience from *The Economist*.) But widespread peer acceptance, and now the Nobel prize, have eluded him. He has taken a typically defiant stance. To voice his recent disappointment, he took out several full-page advertisements in the *Washington Post*, the *New York Times*, and a Swedish newspaper, *Dagens Nyheter*, after the announcement was made. He called on the Nobel committee "to correct its error" and asks Dr Lauterbur and Dr Mansfield to share the prize with him. So far, his demands have fallen on deaf ears.

More Controversy Ahead

The question of who deserves credit for MRI comes down to how you value the crucial steps in invention. John Gore, who directs the Institute of Imaging Science at Vanderbilt University, believes Dr Damadian's abrasive behaviour and outrageous claims may have clouded people's judgment. Since the Nobel committee rewards scientific achievement, not good manners, it would have been fairer to include Dr Damadian in this year's prize. "There is a case to be made that he was a visionary and proposed the idea of scanning through the human body," he says. But Ian Young, an electric engineer at Imperial College in London, and a former colleague of Dr Gore in the EMI/Hammersmith collaboration, disagrees. The "key invention" that everybody uses in MRI today, he says, "is the gradient field."

While another Nobel prize may be awarded for MRI some day, few expect it will be to Dr Damadian. Functional MRI, based on a technique called "blood oxygen level dependent" scanning, a phrase coined by Seiji Ogawa of Bell Labs in 1990 and based on a discovery by Nobel Laureate Linus Pauling and his colleague Charles Coryell, is revolutionising studies of the brain. Like hydrogen nuclei in water, iron in deoxygenated blood acts like a tiny magnet. Because neural activity causes changes in blood oxygenation, researchers can now pinpoint active areas in the brain while people complete various mental activities.

In the early 1990s, a race ensued to create the first human images using this new technique. After being rejected by leading scientific journals because their papers supposedly contained nothing new, two pioneering teams, one from Massachusetts General Hospital in Boston, the other headed by Kamil Ugurbil from the University of Minnesota with Dr Ogawa, successfully submitted papers to the *Proceedings of the National Academy of Sciences*. Both were accepted within days of each other and published in consecutive issues in 1992.

The development of functional MRI mirrors some of the key points that propelled the early development of MRI in the 1970s—the involvement of visionary scientists, strong competition between research teams, and a willingness to challenge accepted notions in the field. The existence of two rival teams suggests that there could be another Nobel dilemma in the making. But with little sign of animosity between the teams, no one expects to see advertisements in the papers when the next prize is awarded.

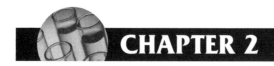

CHAPTER 2

Principal Types of Medical Imaging

Medical Imaging: An Overview of Techniques

By Tamar Nordenberg

Medical imaging has come a long way since the discovery of X-rays in 1895. In the following selection Tamar Nordenberg, a writer for the U.S. Food and Drug Administration's publication *FDA Consumer*, presents an overview of the many uses of X-rays and other imaging technologies. Until late in the twentieth century, conventional X-rays, she explains, were the major tool for detecting everything from tooth decay to breast cancer to bone injuries. However, as Nordenberg explains, conventional X-rays have been supplemented by computed tomography, a technique that combines shots from many different angles into a detailed image. New technologies such as ultrasound and magnetic resonance imaging have also been developed. Ultrasound forms pictures by tracking the echoes of high-pitched sound waves in the body; magnetic resonance creates images using radio waves to detect changes in magnetic polarity. Each type of imaging has particular advantages. Computed tomography has proven useful in identifying tumors in many parts of the body. Magnetic resonance is especially good at imaging the brain and spinal cord as well as blood flow. Ultrasound permits harmless imaging of a developing fetus. Where these are insufficient, other options, such as positron emission tomography, which involves injecting and tracking a radioactive substance in the body, are available. Tamar Nordenberg is a freelance journalist who formerly served as a staff writer for *FDA Consumer.*

ithin a year of German scientist Wilhelm Roentgen's discovery of x-rays in 1895, people throughout the world knew about Roentgen's work and had seen his first x-ray picture—his wife Bertha's hand, showing her bones, wedding ring, and all. Even before Roentgen was awarded the first Nobel Prize in physics in 1901 for his discovery, x-ray studios were popping up that sold bone portraits for display in the home.

As their popularity grew, some publications contained inflated claims about x-rays—they could restore vision to the blind, they could raise the dead. Other people expressed a far more skeptical view: "I can see no future in the field," the head of one x-ray clinic reportedly proclaimed. "All the bones of the body and foreign bodies have been demonstrated."

But x-ray was far from a dead-end technology. Instead, it marked the start of a revolution in medical diagnosis. Like other medical imaging technologies that followed, including ultrasound, computed tomography (or CT) scanning, and magnetic resonance imaging (or MRI), x-ray can help doctors narrow down the causes of a patient's symptoms without surgery and sometimes diagnose an illness before symptoms even appear. While it can't help a blind person see again, used appropriately, medical imaging can be a useful first step in treating a range of problems, from a simple broken bone to a cancerous tumor.

Using medical imaging appropriately, explains William Sacks, M.D., a medical officer in the Food and Drug Administration's radiology branch, means always considering the risks from a device along with its benefits. X-rays and some other imaging tests use radiation, after all, which can have serious health consequences if used improperly. FDA looks at both the risk and benefit sides of the equation to decide whether to allow marketing of a device, Sacks says. And doctors judge the risks versus the benefits in deciding if a test is medically necessary.

FDA, the U.S. Environmental Protection Agency, and other federal and state agencies share the responsibility for protecting the public from unnecessary radiation. For its part, FDA regulates x-ray equipment and all other electronic radiation-emitting products (including nonmedical consumer products, such as microwave ovens) under the Radiation Control for Health and Safety Act. For all electronic imaging devices, the agency develops and enforces standards to ensure that only safe and effective devices are allowed to be marketed.

"Nothing is entirely safe, of course, including walking down the sidewalk," Sacks says. "The question to ask is, 'In balance, do the benefits of x-ray outweigh the safety concerns?' The benefit of making bone portraits for display, like they did at the beginning of the century, is near zero. Now that we know the health risks from certain doses of radiation, we don't order x-rays willy-nilly, but only if there is a health reason to find out something imaging is capable of telling us."

The Many Uses of X-Ray Imaging

Roentgen labeled the rays he discovered with the scientific symbol "X," meaning unknown, because he didn't understand their makeup at first. X-rays are actually electromagnetic waves. When they are passed through a patient's body to a photographic film on the other side, they create a picture of internal body structures called a radiograph.

Chest radiographs, which are among the most common imaging tests, can reveal abnormalities of the lungs (such as pneumonia, tumor or fluid), heart (such as congestive heart failure or enlarged heart), and rib cage (such as broken or abnormal bones).

Other common types of x-ray examinations include dental studies to detect cavities and other tooth and gum problems; abdominal studies, which can reveal abnormalities of not just the abdomen, but also the liver, spleen, gallbladder, and kidneys; gastrointestinal studies of the upper or lower GI tract; studies of the joints to assess things like arthritis and sports injuries; and mammograms, which can help detect breast cancer with the use of special x-ray equipment.

Getting a radiograph takes only a few minutes, at a doctor's office or a radiology unit of a hospital or separate location. After positioning the patient with the body part to be examined between the unit that emits the rays and an x-ray film cassette, the doctor or technician steps away from the area and presses a button or otherwise activates the x-ray machine to take the picture.

The less dense a structure of the body is, the more radiation passes through it and reaches the film. The x-rays expose the film, changing its color after it is developed to gray or black, much like light would darken photographic film.

Bones, as well as tumors, are more dense than soft tissues. They appear white or light on the x-ray film because they absorb much of the radiation, leaving the film only slightly exposed. Structures that are less solid than bone, such as skin, fat, muscles, blood vessels, and the lungs, intestines, and other organs, appear darker on

the film because they let more of the x-rays pass through. Likewise, a break in a bone allows the x-ray beams to pass through, so
the break appears as a dark line in the otherwise white bone.

To make certain organs stand out more clearly, a "contrast
medium"—a substance that blocks x-rays rather than transmitting
any—can be introduced into the body, in the form of a drink or injection. Barium sulfate is commonly used to study the gastrointestinal tract, while iodine-containing dyes are often used to provide information about the gallbladder, kidneys, blood vessels
(using a technique called angiography), or the cavities of the heart.

FDA regulates these contrast agent drugs to make sure they are
safe for patients and helpful in diagnosing their medical condition.

Weighing the Risks

Because x-rays are a type of radiation, patients sometimes express
concerns that the test may harm them somehow, perhaps increase
their risk of cancer. It's true that overexposure to x-rays can damage or destroy living tissue, potentially causing skin burns and
even cancer. But for typical diagnostic x-rays, patient exposure is
"minimal," Sacks says.

Experts estimate that a person in the United States gets only 20
percent of their radiation exposure, on average, from medical x-
rays and other man-made sources. The remaining 80 percent
comes from natural—and usually unavoidable—sources, such as
radon gas, the human body, outer space, and rocks and soil.

Many factors affect a person's actual dose of radiation each
year. One of the most influential factors is the elevation of a person's home town. The higher the elevation, the thinner the atmos-
phere and the greater one's exposure to cosmic radiation from
outer space. At sea level, FDA's Sacks explains, a person typically
gets about two chest x-rays' worth of cosmic radiation each year.
That amount can be significantly higher, he says, in high-altitude
cities like Denver or Santa Fe.

Particularly over the last two decades, improvements in x-ray
technology have meant decreasing patient exposure to radiation.
Not as high a dose of radiation is needed to get a useful diagnostic image, and the rays can be focused more precisely on the part
of the body to be studied.

Still, some precautions are taken to make the x-ray procedure
even safer. For example, a lead apron sometimes is placed over

those parts of the body not being studied, especially the reproductive organs, which are extrasensitive to radiation. Because radiation exposure can cause birth defects to a fetus in certain stages of development, pregnant women should get x-rays only when absolutely needed, and a lead apron should be used to shield the mother and fetus when possible.

Introducing Computed Tomography

Unlike conventional x-rays, which take a single picture of a part of the body, an updated version of the technology called computed tomography generates hundreds of x-ray images in a single examination. Despite the large number of images, the total amount of radiation can be less from a 30- to 45-minute CT scan than from some conventional x-ray procedures.

The patient lies still on an examination table that slides into a circular opening in the CT scanner. The x-ray tube that surrounds the patient takes the pictures from many different directions, and then a computer takes the images and constructs them into two-dimensional cross sections of the body, which can be viewed on a television screen.

"There was nothing uncomfortable about the test, nothing to be afraid of," says Wanda Diak, the managing director of a support network called CancerHope, who underwent several CT scans in 1996 and '97 to track the status of her ovarian cancer.

Computed tomography produces detailed images that can sometimes reveal abnormalities an ordinary x-ray would not pick up. CT scanning can be useful in checking the brain for tumors, aneurysms, bleeding, or other abnormalities. Also, it can unveil tumors, cysts, or other problems in the liver, spleen, pancreas, lungs, kidneys, pelvis, lymph glands, and other body parts. . . .

Magnetic Resonance Imaging

First cleared for marketing in 1984, magnetic resonance imaging [MRI], like x-ray and CT scanning, provides a look inside the body without surgery. MRI differs in a basic respect from its predecessor technologies, however: MRI uses a strong magnetic field, not x-rays, to create a picture of the internal body structure being studied.

Typically, during MRI, the patient lies on a table that slides into a tubular scanner for the 30- to 90-minute test. Patients are often given earphones to wear while inside the tunnel to block out the loud clanking noises the machine makes.

Inside the tube, a large, donut-shaped magnet creates a magnetic field. Pulse radio waves are directed into the magnetic field and absorbed by hydrogen atoms in the body. The machine's computers create an image of the body's internal structure by measuring the emission of energy from the movement of hydrogen atoms within the patient's body.

MRI is especially useful in studying the brain and spinal cord, the soft tissues of the body, and the joints. Because this technique shows distinct contrast between normal and abnormal tissues, it is sometimes superior to CT scanning and other imaging methods in evaluating tumors, tissue damage, and blood flow.

MRI scanning has no known long-term risks. No jewelry or other metal can be carried or worn during the exam, though, because of the very strong magnetic field. Most importantly, the health professional overseeing the treatment must be told if a patient has a pacemaker, hearing aid, any metal implants such as artificial joints, plates, or screws, or other metal implants or electrical devices. The magnet could interfere with these devices and cause serious injury, even death in the case of a pacemaker.

While MRI is a painless procedure, people who tend to feel claustrophobic may be uncomfortable inside the tunnel. For those people, anti-anxiety medicines are available, or they may choose a hospital or clinic that offers the less confining "open MRI" machine.

Variety of Ultrasound Applications

Ultrasound scanning isn't just for viewing a developing fetus, anymore. Originally used for this purpose, ultrasound today substitutes for conventional x-rays in the diagnosis of many conditions, commonly those involving the kidneys, bladder and uterus, the heart (called echocardiography), and the spleen, gallbladder and pancreas. However, ultrasound does not produce clear images of the lungs and other organs filled with gas or air.

With an ultrasound exam, a gel is spread over the skin covering the area of interest, and a "transducer" is moved back and forth to gather data. The transducer sends out high-frequency sound waves, far above the range of human hearing. When the waves hit the body part being studied, some are absorbed by tissues, and some are echoed back to a transducer. The machine measures the amount of sound reflected back, and displays an image called a sonogram on a monitor or on videotape or graph paper.

An ultrasound exam can take anywhere from 15 minutes to an hour.

While ultrasound is considered risk-free, FDA's Sacks says it still should be used only when medically warranted because "[t]here's no point in taking a chance for anything but a medical reason."

Choosing the Right Imaging Technique

So, which diagnostic imaging technique is best? "Best for what? It really depends what you're looking for," says board-certified diagnostic radiologist Mark E. Klein, M.D. He likens the question to asking which mode of transportation is best: "In the mountains, you'd want a helicopter or four-wheel drive. On ice, you'd want a Zamboni." For example, he says, a skull x-ray to look for a brain lesion is useless, so the best choice might be a CT scan or MRI. For a broken arm, an x-ray would do the job and is preferred over an MRI.

X-ray, CT scanning, MRI, and ultrasound are among the most common noninvasive procedures (or minimally invasive, in some cases when a contrast agent is used), but the diagnostic options don't end there. Nuclear scanning, including two techniques called positron emission tomography (PET) and single photon emission computed tomography (SPECT), use radioactive substances introduced into the body to discern abnormal from normal body structures or evaluate the body's functioning. Other, sometimes riskier procedures require the insertion of tubes or instruments into the body.

A patient should know why the doctor is choosing a certain imaging technique, Sacks says. "The patient ought to feel secure about what's being done and understand the doctor's reasoning: 'What information does the doctor expect to get from this test?'"

During the test, too, the technician or radiologist can help the patient feel more secure. Julie (who asked that her last name not be used) says she didn't feel upset or panicky during her MRIs in 1997 to follow her uterine cancer. "The technicians were very careful to help me understand what to expect and what I would feel—10 seconds of this, a minute of that, hold still for this length of time. I felt thoroughly prepared for it."

Her last MRI confirmed that she was "all clean" of cancer.

"Even if the tests revealed bad news, I'm very thrilled they were there to give doctors a good view of my situation."

Wanda Diak's ovarian cancer has not been evident for almost three years. During her follow-up exams, she says, her doctor sometimes taps on her stomach to check for signs of recurrence. The method seemed primitive to Diak, but her doctor pointed out that before CT scans and other imaging, different sounds were all doctors had to clue them in to an abnormality.

"I think about someone tapping on your stomach rather than having this image that essentially slices you in half so you can see inside," Diak says. "Its like the caveman to the year 2000."

Conventional X-Rays and Radiation

By the National Institutes of Health

According to the National Institutes of Health in the following selection, the discovery of X-rays in 1895 enabled physicians to "see"
inside the body for the first time, greatly enhancing disease diagnosis. However, shortly after the discovery, scientists learned that
X-rays were not an unmitigated good. Researchers realized that high-
intensity radiation, such as that produced by X-ray machines, could
cause cancer in those exposed to it. However, the National Institutes
of Health explains that as X-ray equipment and procedures have improved, patients receive much lower doses of radiation than in the
past and are therefore at less risk of getting cancer. Moreover, physicians are careful to use X-rays only when necessary. Founded in
1887, the National Institutes of Health comprise the federal government's leading medical research bodies.

We live in a sea of radiation. There are many different types
of radiation, some of which are visible light, ultraviolet
rays from the sun, infrared from a heat lamp, mi-
crowaves, radio waves and ionizing radiation. Radiation is said to
be ionizing if it has sufficient energy to displace one or more of
the electrons that are part of an atom. This creates an electrically
charged atom known as an ion. Common examples of ionizing radiation are x rays, which are generated by machines, and gamma
rays, which are emitted by radioactive materials. Others include
alpha and beta rays, which are also emitted from radioactive materials, and neutrons, which are emitted during the splitting (fis-
sion) of atoms in a nuclear reactor.

National Institutes of Health, "What We Know About Radiation, www.nih.gov, April 2000.

Encountering Ionizing Radiation

Everyone who lives on this planet is constantly exposed to naturally occurring ionizing radiation (background radiation). This has been true since the dawn of time. The average effective dose equivalent of radiation to which a person in the United States is exposed annually is estimated to be about 350 millirem. (A millirem is a unit that estimates the biological impact of a particular type of radiation absorbed in the body.)

Sources of background radiation include cosmic rays from the sun and stars; naturally occurring radioactive materials in rocks and soil; radionuclides (unstable radioactive counterparts to naturally stable atoms) normally incorporated into our body's tissues; and radon and its products, which we inhale. Radon exists as a gas and is present in soil from which it seeps into the air. Radon gets trapped inside buildings, especially if the ventilation is poor. Levels of environmental radiation depend upon geology, how we construct our dwellings, and altitude. For example, radiation levels from cosmic rays are greater for people on airplanes and those living on the Colorado plateau. This low-level background radiation is a part of the earth's natural environment and any degree of risk associated with it has not been demonstrated to date.

We are also exposed to ionizing radiation from man-made sources, mostly through medical procedures. On the average, doses from a diagnostic x ray are much lower, in dose effective terms, than natural background radiation. Radiation therapy, however, can reach levels many times higher than background radiation but this is usually targeted only to the affected tissues. Besides extremely small amounts of ionizing radiation from color televisions and smoke detectors, there are small amounts of ionizing radiation in many building materials and mining and agricultural products, such as granite, coal, and potassium salt. People who smoke receive additional radiation from radionuclides in tobacco smoke.

The Effects of Large Doses of Ionizing Radiation

The adverse effects of large doses of radiation were seen shortly after the discovery of radioactivity and x rays in the 1890s. In 1902, skin cancers were reported in scientists who were studying radioactivity. Back then, no one took special precautions in working with radioactive materials because their effects were not yet fully recognized. The occupational hazards soon became apparent. For example, the widely publicized reports on radium dial painters described cases of bone cancer in women who wet their brushes on their tongues to get a good "point" for painting radium on watch dials. The role of radiation in causing leukemia in humans was first reported in 1944 in physicians and radiologists.

Much of our data on the effects of large doses of radiation comes from survivors of the 1945 atomic bombs dropped on Hiroshima and Nagasaki and from other people who received large doses of radiation, usually for treatment. The National Cancer Institute (NCI, part of the National Institutes of Health (NIH), in collaboration with the Radiation Effects Research Foundation, an international group supported jointly by the U.S. Department of Energy and the Japanese Ministry of Health and Welfare, continues to study the long-term effects of radiation on the survivors of the bombs. The percentage of cancers related to radiation depends on the dose received; on the average, only about 12% of all the cancers that have developed among those survivors who were studied are estimated to be related to radiation; only about 9% of the fatal cancers in this study population are estimated to be related to radiation.

Other populations exposed to radioactive materials are also being studied. Uranium miners who were exposed to radon in the mines and those who lived near the Nevada nuclear weapons test site that was used from 1951 to 1963 and who experienced fallout from the atmospheric tests have been evaluated. NCI also is working with the ministries of health of Belarus and Ukraine to set up studies of the children most affected by the 1986 Chernobyl nuclear power plant accident and of the workers who cleaned up the plant after the accident. The information from all these studies has been and will continue to be published—after rigorous review— in medical and scientific journals that are available to everyone. . . .

X Rays Use Radiation to Benefit Patients

The discovery of x rays in 1895 was a major turning point in diagnosing diseases because physicians finally had an easy way to "see" inside the body without having to operate. . . .

The use of ionizing radiation has led to major improvements in the diagnosis and treatment of patients with cancer. These innovations have resulted in increased survival rates and improved quality of life. Mammography can detect breast cancer at an early stage when it may be curable. Needle biopsies are more safe, accurate, and informative when guided by x ray or other imaging techniques. . . .

Radiation's Effects

Ionizing radiation can cause important changes in our cells by breaking the electron bonds that hold molecules together. For example, radiation can damage our genetic material (deoxyribonucleic acid or DNA) either directly by displacing electrons from the DNA molecule, or indirectly by displacing electrons from some other molecule in the cell that then interacts with the DNA. A cell can be destroyed quickly or its growth or function may be altered through a change (or mutation) that may not be evident for many years. However, the possibility of this inducing a clinically significant illness or other problem is quite remote at small radiation doses.

Our cells, however, have several mechanisms to repair the damage done to DNA by radiation. The efficiency of these repair mechanisms differs among cells and depends on several things, including the type and dose of radiation. There also are biological factors that can greatly modify the cancer-causing effects of large doses of radiation.

The severity of radiation's effects depends on many other factors such as the magnitude and duration of the dose; the area of the body exposed to it; and a person's sex, age, and physical condition. A very large dose of radiation to the whole body at one time can result in death. Exposure to large doses of radiation can increase the risk of developing cancer. Because a radiation-induced cancer is indistinguishable from cancer caused by other factors, it is very difficult to pinpoint radiation as the cause of cancer in a particular individual.

Other effects of large doses of radiation include suppression of the immune system and cataracts. Certain tissues of a fetus, particularly the brain, are especially sensitive to radiation at specific stages of development. However, the children and grandchildren of the atomic bomb survivors so far have shown no greater incidence of genetic problems than do unexposed populations.

It is very difficult to detect biologic effects in animals or people who are exposed to small doses of radiation. Based on studies in animals and in people exposed to large doses of radiation such as the atomic bomb survivors, scientists have made conservative estimates of what might be the largest doses that would be reasonably safe for a person over a lifetime. But these calculations are estimates only, based on mathematical models. Low-level exposures received by the general public have shown no link to cancer induction. Even so, the U.S. Government uses these estimates to set the limits on all potential exposures to radiation for workers in jobs that expose them to ionizing radiation. International experts and various scientific committees have, over the years, examined the massive body of knowledge about radiation effects in developing and refining radiation protection standards.

Patients and Radiation

The doses involved in medical procedures that use radiation or radioactive materials have been decreasing over the past two decades as x ray films and equipment have been improved. Also, the ability to target radiation more precisely to one part of the body has resulted in less exposure to the rest of the body.

It is always wise to avoid unnecessary radiation exposure. Physicians routinely compare the risks of radiation to the benefits derived from a diagnostic use of radiation to ensure that there is more benefit to the patient than risk. In many cases, such diagnostic tests enable doctors to treat the patient without invasive and life-threatening procedures.

Radiologists, health physicists, the National Council on Radiation Protection and Measurements—the Congressionally chartered independent advisory group that, among other things, recommends what the U.S. radiation standards should be—and other responsible parties are continually seeking ways of minimizing risk while retaining or improving the benefits from medical uses of radiation.

Therefore, patients should not be concerned about radiation exposure from medical tests as the benefits of these procedures far outweigh the potential risks from their exposure.

Computed Tomography

By Conall J. Garvey and Rebecca Hanlon

Computed tomography, better known as CT or CAT scan (Computed Axial Tomography), has been in use for several decades now. The technology represents a major advance in the use of X-rays to image internal organs. In the following selection two British radiology specialists describe how the technology works and how it is used in medical practice. Conventional X-ray images show a two-dimensional picture of the entire three-dimensional area under examination. Everything inside is squashed down into a single image. That means, for example, a bone might mask a tumor that lies under it. Tomography enables technicians to obtain an X-ray image of a particular plane through the body. In a CT scan the X-ray transmitter rotates around the patient's body, as do detectors on the opposite side. With the aid of computers, a series of narrow-section images is assembled into complete "slice" image of the head or body. The computer can also stack the slices to create a three-dimensional picture.

In its early days, the authors report, CT scanning had several drawbacks. One was that the power cables prevented a complete rotation of the X-ray ring around the body. Also, the process was slow and prone to distortion because of the patient's breathing or movement. But an innovation in power-cable connections and a new technique called spiral scanning have made scans easier and faster. Another significant innovation is the multislice scanner, which snaps several different planes at once, thanks to multiple detector arrays opposite the X-ray source. The authors state that CT scans are preferable to magnetic resonance images in certain situations, such as when doctors need images of head or pelvis injuries.

Conall J. Garvey is a consultant radiologist at the Royal Liverpool University Hospital in the United Kingdom. Rebecca Hanlon is a specialist registrar in radiology at the same institution.

Conall J. Garvey and Rebecca Hanlon, "Computed Tomography in Clinical Practice," *British Medical Journal,* vol. 324, May 4, 2002, pp. 1,077–80. Copyright © 2002 by the British Medical Association. Reproduced by permission.

Computed tomography was first introduced 30 years ago and has since become an integral part of clinical practice. Because of rapid advances in technology few clinicians are aware of the scope and limitations of the different types of scanners. This review describes the three main types of computed tomographic scanner that are used in routine clinical practice and discusses their use in the investigation of a wide range of different conditions. It also [highlights] differing views on the relative merits of computed tomography versus magnetic resonance imaging.

The information contained in this review was gathered from several sources. These include many years of personal experience using computed tomography and magnetic resonance imaging, discussions with manufacturers of equipment, and knowledge of radiation dosimetry issues, supported by a search of Medline and the Cochrane databases for systematic reviews comparing computed tomography and magnetic resonance imaging.

By today's [2002] standards early computed tomographic scanners were extremely slow and required enormous computer facilities to generate comparatively crude scans. Improvements in tube technology and computer hardware and software have shortened scan times and improved the resolution of scans. The incorporation of slip ring technology into scanners in the late 1980s resulted in the development of spiral (helical) scanners. More recently, multislice scanners with scan times of less than a second have become widely available. These important technological changes have been linked to newer and faster computers to provide the systems that are currently available.

Early CT Scanners

In first generation (conventional) scanners, the tube produces a narrow beam of X-rays that passes through the patient and is picked up by a row of detectors on the other side. The tube and detectors are positioned on opposite sides of a ring that rotates around the patient. The physical linkages between the power cables and the tube mean that the tube is unable to rotate continuously. After each rotation the scanner must stop and rotate in the opposite direction. Each rotation acquires an axial image, typically with a slice thickness of 1 cm, taking approximately 1 second per rotation. The table moves the patient a set distance through the scanner between each slice.

Conventional scanners have some limitations. The scan time is slow, and scans are prone to artefact caused by movement or breathing. Scanners have a poor ability to reformat in different planes, studies of dynamic contrast are impossible, and small lesions between slices may be missed.

Many departments are now acquiring spiral scanners, and it is anticipated that over the next few years half the scanners in the United Kingdom will be multislice scanners. Often a conventional scanner is retained alongside a new scanner. Conventional scanners still have a role, mainly in non-contrast examinations[1] that do not require fast scanning for optimal vascular enhancement. A large bulk of the computed tomography workload of many large radiology departments consists of routine examinations of the head by unenhanced computed tomography—for example, for cerebral infarcts or haemorrhage. These can still be performed satisfactorily on an existing conventional scanner, thus freeing time on the spiral scanner.

Spiral Scanners

The incorporation of slip ring technology into the design of scanners in the late 1980s removed the need for a rigid mechanical linkage between the power cables and the x-ray tube. This "simple" development, by enabling the tube to rotate in one direction indefinitely, has re-established computed tomography at the forefront of imaging. While the tube is rotating, the table supporting the patient also moves continuously so that a volume of tissue rather than individual slices is scanned. The data are then reformatted automatically to display the images as axial slices. High quality reconstructed (reformatted) images in coronal, sagittal, and oblique planes can be readily acquired on a workstation.

Spiral scanning has several advantages. The scan time is much shorter than that of conventional computed tomography. Closely spaced scans are readily obtained, allowing good quality reconstructions in different planes. Lesions can be evaluated during different phases of contrast enhancement. Computed tomographic angiography is possible, and the likelihood that a small lesion may be overlooked is less/smaller. Spiral computed tomography is a powerful diagnostic tool. A spiral scanner is not as fast as a mul-

1. Contrast scans involve the injection of dye into the bloodstream to enhance contrast.

tislice scanner but is considerably cheaper (typically one third to one half the cost of a multislice scanner).

A multislice (multidetector) computed tomographic scanner can be considered as a "turbocharged" spiral scanner. Conventional and spiral scanners use a single row of detectors to pick up the x-ray beam after it has passed through the patient. Multislice scanners currently have up to eight active rows of detectors, and scanners under development will use direct digital detectors on flat panels (GE Medical Systems, personal communication). The increased number of detectors and tube rotation times that take a fraction of a second combine to give faster coverage of a given volume of tissue. Newer multislice scanners also come with faster computer software, offering increased reconstruction and post-processing capabilities.

The use of a four row scanner offers various options to the radiologist. A large volume of the patient can be scanned during a single breath hold (for example, thorax, abdomen, and pelvis in a trauma patient in 20 seconds). Alternatively, a normal volume can be examined by using much finer slices (for example, acquisition of 1 mm sections through the chest in 20 seconds, improving detail and facilitating reformatted images of better quality). In theory, the time taken to perform a scan with a multislice scanner with four detectors would be a quarter of that of a single slice spiral scanner. In practice, a multislice scanner acquires images two to three times faster than a single slice scanner.

Use of a multislice scanner will considerably increase [the flow] of patients compared with a conventional scanner, but the [flow] will be similar to that achieved with a modern spiral scanner. Multislice scanners generate an increased amount of data compared with single slice scanners, and in practice the throughput of patients is limited by the time taken to image and reconstruct these data. For institutions with a picture archive and communication system (PACS, the "filmless hospital"), the volume of data resulting from studies of multislice computed tomography can pose considerable strain on storage systems. If more patients are scanned and more information acquired during each examination the radiologists' workload will significantly increase.

X-ray tubes are expensive. In the United Kingdom in 2002, a typical spiral scanner can expect to have one tube replaced per year at a cost of £300,000–400,000 [$550,000–$750,000]. The life of the tube for a multislice scanner should be the same as the tube for a single slice scanner if the same techniques are used. Since many patients examined on a multislice scanner will have multi-phase and fine slice studies, the tube life may be shorter, requiring more regular replacement.

Higher Radiation Doses

Computed tomography accounts for 40% of medical diagnostic radiation [absorbed by patients] but represents only 4% of radiology examinations. Any expansion in the use of computed tomography will need to be balanced against the radiation dose. Readers are referred to the guidelines published and regularly upgraded by the Royal College of Radiologists.

The views whether multislice scanners will lead to an increase or decrease in population dose from examinations by computed tomography differ. Generally the dose from a multislice spiral scanner is slightly greater than from a single slice spiral scanner. Because multislice scanners are faster, more slices tend to be performed and more images acquired in different phases of enhancement, which results in an increased dose of radiation. In 1992, the National Radiological Protection Board pointed out the potential for high doses to patients from inappropriate examinations by computed tomography. More recently, the U.S. Food and Drug Administration raised the alarm about the dangers of unnecessary scans and excessive radiation. Particular concerns were raised about the use of computed tomography in children and patients of small stature and the increasing use of the technique for screening for lung cancer and cardiac artery disease.

Computed tomography is a highly useful tool for solving problems. It should, however, never be allowed to replace proper history taking and clinical examination. Radiologists must use their knowledge to ensure that requests for computed tomography are appropriate and use low dose protocols targeted at the clinical problem.

Comparison with Magnetic Resonance

The lack of systematic reviews comparing magnetic resonance imaging and computed tomography is notable. A search of the Cochrane database found no complete reviews and only a small number of quality assessed systematic reviews. In our view, many radiologists practising the two techniques are rivals. On the positive side, this rivalry has been responsible for many innovations, but it may encourage proponents to advocate their particular technique in a biased fashion. This, combined with a dearth of high quality systematic reviews, could lead to confusion among clinicians when trying to determine which investigation is most appropriate for a given condition.

In general, magnetic resonance is excellent for imaging soft tissue and bone marrow. It is not generally used in patients with acute trauma, in the evaluation of the lungs, or in the assessment of cortical bone. Currently, most studies by magnetic resonance imaging take much longer than a spiral or multislice scan of the same area. Computed tomography is generally better for examinations of areas prone to motion, such as the lungs and the bowel. Availability of scanner time and cost are the major limiting factors for magnetic resonance imaging, whereas radiation dose and potential nephrotoxicity from iodinated contrast agents are the limiting factors for computed tomography.

Computed tomography remains the primary imaging technique for acute cranial trauma, but for most other cerebral applications magnetic resonance imaging has superseded computed tomography. In the abdomen, computed tomography is generally superior to magnetic resonance imaging for the hollow viscera. Examination of the solid organs is more contentious. State of the art computed tomography and magnetic resonance imaging are competitive for liver, spleen, kidneys, and possibly pancreas. Magnetic resonance imaging is superior for the pelvic organs. Which test to perform will be influenced by local expertise, availability of equipment, cost, and radiation dose.

Spiral scanning has enabled the development of computed tomographic fluoroscopy, providing real time imaging for intervention procedures guided by computed tomography. For example, when percutaneous lung biopsies are performed the needle can be guided in through the lung under direct vision. This means that the track of the needle can be constantly adjusted so that it is in line with the target area. In theory the number of punctures to the lung could be lowered appreciably, thus reducing the time of the procedure and the discomfort to the patient.

Magnetic resonance imaging has a limited role in patients with major trauma and in patients on ventilators because of the challenge posed by the magnetic environment to anaesthetics and monitoring of patients. Contraindications for magnetic resonance imaging include pacemakers and certain metallic implants.

Most units that perform magnetic resonance imaging report a failure rate of 3–6% as a result of patients' claustrophobia or inability to keep still during the long scanning times, particularly in young or elderly patients. Primary care doctors often have to reassure patients who are anxious about undergoing magnetic resonance imaging. As the technology improves, scanners are becoming faster and, with the introduction of "open" magnets and dedicated extremity magnets, claustrophobia may become a thing of the past.

Multislice computed tomography, with its speed and capability of multiplanar reformats, can be substituted for magnetic resonance imaging in several clinical situations. But if magnetic resonance imaging is indicated as the first line investigation then this is preferable because of the lack of ionising [potentially harmful] radiation.

Magnetic Resonance Imaging

By Kurt Richard Sternlof

Magnetic resonance imaging (MRI) uses strong magnets and radio waves to create images of the body's interior, explains Kurt Richard Sternlof in the following selection. It is more sensitive than other imaging techniques such as X-rays, he says, and is often used to more fully investigate negative results from other tests. According to Sternlof, an MRI can be used to diagnose problems all over the body, including inside the brain, bones, and joints, and the circulatory system. The procedure has no known risks, except for people with metal objects in their bodies, he notes, and normally requires no aftercare. The procedure simply requires the patient to lie still in an MRI tube for approximately thirty to ninety minutes. Sternlof is a science writer from New Rochelle, New York.

Magnetic resonance imaging (MRI) is one of the newest, and perhaps most versatile, medical imaging technologies available. Doctors can get highly refined images of the body's interior without surgery using MRI. By using strong magnets and pulses of radio waves to manipulate the natural magnetic properties in the body, this technique makes better images of organs and soft tissues than those of other brain scanning technologies. MRI is particularly useful for imaging the brain and spine, as well as the soft tissues of joints and the interior structure of bones, as well as the liver. The entire body is visible with MRI, and the technique poses few known health risks.

MRI was developed in the 1980s. Its technology has been developed for use in magnetic resonance angiography (MRA), magnetic resonance spectroscopy (MRS), and, more recently, magnetic resonance cholangiopancreatography (MRCP). MRA was developed to study blood flow, whereas MRS can identify the chemical composition of diseased tissue and produce color images of brain function. MRCP is evolving into a potential noninvasive alternative for the diagnostic procedure endoscopic retrograde cholangiopancreatography (ERCP).[1]

Advantages of MRI

MRI creates precise images of the body based on the varying proportions of magnetic elements in different tissues. Very minor fluctuations in chemical composition can be determined. MRI images have greater natural contrast than standard x rays, computed tomography scan (CT scan), or ultrasound, all of which depend on the differing physical properties of tissues. This sensitivity allows MRI to distinguish fine variations in tissues deep within the body. It is also particularly useful for spotting and distinguishing diseased tissues (tumors and other lesions) early in their development. Often, doctors prescribe an MRI scan to more fully investigate earlier findings of other imaging techniques.

The entire body can be scanned, from head to toe and from the skin to the deepest recesses of the brain. Moreover, MRI scans are not obstructed by bone, gas, or body waste, which can hinder other imaging techniques. (Although the scans can be degraded by motion such as breathing, heartbeat, and bowel activity.) The MRI process produces cross-sectional images of the body that are as sharp in the middle as on the edges, even of the brain through the skull. A close series of these two-dimensional images can provide a three-dimensional view of the targeted area. Along with images from the cross-sectional plane, the MRI can also provide images sagitally (from one side of the body to the other, from left to right for example), allowing for a better three-dimensional interpretation, which is sometimes very important for planning a surgical approach.

MRI does not depend on potentially harmful ionizing radiation, as do standard x ray and computer tomography scans. There are no known risks specific to the procedure, other than for people who might have metal objects in their bodies.

---

1. a procedure that enables the diagnosis of problems in the liver, gallbladder, bile ducts, and pancreas

Despite its many advantages, MRI is not routinely used because it is a somewhat complex and costly procedure. MRI requires large, expensive, and complicated equipment; a highly trained operator; and a doctor specializing in radiology. Generally, MRI is prescribed only when serious symptoms or negative results from other tests indicate a need. Many times another test is appropriate for the type of diagnosis needed.

Uses

Doctors may prescribe an MRI scan of different areas of the body.

Brain and head

MRI technology was developed because of the need for brain imaging. It is one of the few imaging tools that can see through bone (the skull) and deliver high quality pictures of the brain's delicate soft tissue structures. MRI may be needed for patients with symptoms of a brain tumor, stroke, or infection (like meningitis). MRI may also be needed when cognitive or psychological symptoms suggest brain disease (like Alzheimer's or Huntington's diseases, or multiple sclerosis), or when developmental retardation suggests a birth defect. MRI can also provide pictures of the sinuses and other areas of the head beneath the face. In adult and pediatric patients, MRI may be better able to detect abnormalities than compared to computed tomography scanning.

Spine

Spinal problems can create a host of seemingly unrelated symptoms. MRI is particularly useful for identifying and evaluating degenerated or herniated spinal discs. It can also be used to determine the condition of nerve tissue within the spinal cord.

Joint

MRI scanning is most commonly used to diagnose and assess joint problems. MRI can provide clear images of the bone, cartilage, ligament, and tendon that comprise a joint. MRI can be used to diagnose joint injuries due to sports, advancing age, or arthritis. MRI can also be used to diagnose shoulder problems, such as a torn rotator cuff. MRI can also detect the presence of an otherwise hidden tumor or infection in a joint, and can be used to diagnose the nature of developmental joint abnormalities in children.

Skeleton

The properties of MRI that allow it to see through the skull also allow it to view the inside of bones. Accordingly, it can be used to detect bone cancer, inspect the marrow for leukemia and other diseases, assess bone loss (osteoporosis), and examine complex fractures.

Heart and circulation

MRI technology can be used to evaluate the circulatory system. The heart and blood flow provides a good natural contrast medium that allows structures of the heart to be clearly distinguished.

The rest of the body.

Whereas computed tomography and ultrasound scans satisfy most chest, abdominal, and general body imaging needs, MRI may be needed in certain circumstances to provide better pictures or when repeated scanning is required. The progress of some therapies, like liver cancer therapy, needs to be monitored, and the effect of repeated x-ray exposure is a concern.

MRI Scans and Metal

MRI scanning should not be used when there is the potential for an interaction between the strong MRI magnet and metal objects that might be imbedded in a patient's body. The force of magnetic attraction on certain types of metal objects (including surgical steel) could move them within the body and cause serious injury. Metal may be imbedded in a person's body for several reasons.

People with implanted cardiac pacemakers, metal aneurysm clips, or who have broken bones repaired with metal pins, screws, rods, or plates must tell their radiologist prior to having an MRI scan. In some cases (like a metal rod in a reconstructed leg), the difficulty may be overcome.

Patients must tell their doctor if they have bullet fragments or other metal pieces in their body from old wounds. The suspected presence of metal, whether from an old or recent wound, should be confirmed before scanning.

People with significant work exposure to metal particles (e.g., working with a metal grinder) should discuss this with their doctor and radiologist. The patient may need prescan testing—usually a single, regular x ray of the eyes to see if any metal is present. . . .

Side Effects

The potential side effects of magnetic and electric fields on human health remain a source of debate. In particular, the possible effects on an unborn baby are not well known. Any woman who is, or may be, pregnant, should carefully discuss this issue with her doctor and radiologist before undergoing a scan.

As with all medical imaging techniques, obesity greatly interferes with the quality of MRI.

Mapping Hydrogen

In essence, MRI produces a map of hydrogen distribution in the body. Hydrogen is the simplest element known, the most abundant in biological tissue, and one that can be magnetized. It will align itself within a strong magnetic field, like the needle of a compass. The earth's magnetic field is not strong enough to keep a person's hydrogen atoms pointing in the same direction, but the superconducting magnet of an MRI machine can. This comprises the magnetic part of MRI.

Once a patient's hydrogen atoms have been aligned in the magnet, pulses of very specific radio wave frequencies are used to knock them back out of alignment. The hydrogen atoms alternately absorb and emit radio wave energy, vibrating back and forth between their resting (magnetized) state and their agitated (radio pulse) state. This comprises the resonance part of MRI.

The MRI equipment records the duration, strength, and source location of the signals emitted by the atoms as they relax and translates the data into an image on a television monitor. The state of hydrogen in diseased tissue differs from healthy tissue of the same type, making MRI particularly good at identifying tumors and other lesions. In some cases, chemical agents . . . can be injected to improve the contrast between healthy and diseased tissue.

A single MRI exposure produces a two-dimensional image of a slice through the entire target area. A series of these image slices closely spaced (usually less than half an inch) makes a virtual three-dimensional view of the area.

Other Uses of MRI Technology

Magnetic resonance spectroscopy (MRS) is different from MRI because MRS uses a continuous band of radio wave frequencies to excite hydrogen atoms in a variety of chemical compounds other than water. These compounds absorb and emit radio energy at characteristic frequencies, or spectra, which can be used to identify them. Generally, a color image is created by assigning a color to each distinctive spectral emission. This comprises the spectroscopy part of MRS. MRS is still experimental and is available only in a few research centers.

Doctors primarily use MRS to study the brain and disorders like epilepsy, Alzheimer's disease, brain tumors, and the effects of drugs on brain growth and metabolism. The technique is also useful in evaluating metabolic disorders of the muscles and nervous system.

Magnetic resonance angiography (MRA) is another variation on standard MRI. MRA, like other types of angiography, looks specifically at fluid flow within the blood (vascular) system, but does so without the injection of dyes or radioactive tracers. Standard MRI cannot make a good picture of flowing blood, but MRA uses specific radio pulse sequences to capture usable signals. The technique is generally used in combination with MRI to obtain images that show both vascular structure and flow within the brain and head in cases of stroke, or when a blood clot or aneurysm is suspected.

MRI technology is also being applied in the evaluation of the pancreatic and biliary ducts in a new study called magnetic resonance cholangiopancreatography (MRCP). MRCP produces images similar to that of endoscopic retrograde cholangiopancreatography (ERCP), but in a non-invasive manner. Because MRCP is new and still very expensive, it is not readily available in most hospitals and imaging centers.

The Procedure

Regardless of the exact type of MRI planned, or area of the body targeted, the procedure involved is basically the same. In a special MRI suite, the patient lies down on a narrow table and is made as comfortable as possible. Transmitters are positioned on the body and the table moves into a long tube that houses the magnet. The tube is as long as an average adult lying down, and is open at both ends. Once the area to be examined has been properly positioned, a radio pulse is applied. Then a two-dimensional image corresponding to one slice through the area is made. The table then moves a fraction of an inch and the next image is made. Each image exposure takes several seconds and the entire exam will last anywhere from 30 to 90 minutes. During this time, the patient must remain still as movement can distort the pictures produced.

Depending on the area to be imaged, the radio-wave transmitters will be positioned in different locations.

- For the head and neck, a helmet-like covering is worn on the head.
- For the spine, chest, and abdomen, the patient will be lying on the transmitters.
- For the knee, shoulder, or other joint, the transmitters will be applied directly to the joint.

Additional probes will monitor vital signs (like pulse, respiration, etc.) throughout the test.

The procedure is somewhat noisy and can feel confining to many patients. As the patient moves through the tube, the patient hears a thumping sound. Sometimes, music is supplied via earphones to drown out the noise. Some patients may become anxious or feel claustrophobic while in the small, enclosed tube. Patients may be reassured to know that throughout the study, they can communicate with medical personnel through an intercom-like system.

Recently, open MRIs have become available. Instead of a tube open only at the ends, an open MRI also has opening at the sides. Open MRIs are preferable for patients who have a fear of closed spaces and become anxious in traditional MRI machines. Open MRIs can also better accommodate obese patients, and allow parents to accompany their children during testing.

If the chest or abdomen is to be imaged, the patient will be asked to hold his or her breath as each exposure is made. Other instructions may be given to the patient as needed. In many cases, the entire examination will be performed by an MRI operator who is not a doctor. However, the supervising radiologist should be available to consult as necessary during the exam, and will view and interpret the results sometime later.

Preparation and Aftercare

In some cases (such as for MRI brain scanning or MRA), a chemical designed to increase image contrast may be given immediately before the exam. If a patient suffers from anxiety or claustrophobia, drugs may be given to help the patient relax.

The patient must remove all metal objects (watches, jewelry, eye glasses, hair clips, etc.). Any magnetized objects (like credit and bank machine cards, audio tapes, etc.) should be kept far away from the MRI equipment because they can be erased. The patient cannot bring any personal items such as a wallet or keys into the MRI machine. The patient may be asked to wear clothing without metal snaps, buckles, or zippers, unless a medical gown is worn during the procedure. The patient may be asked not to use hair spray, hair gel, or cosmetics that could interfere with the scan.

No aftercare is necessary, unless the patient received medication or had a reaction to a contrast agent. Normally, patients can immediately return to their daily activities. If the exam reveals a serious condition that requires more testing or treatment, appropriate information and counseling will be needed.

MRI poses no known health risks to the patient and produces no physical side effects. Again, the potential effects of MRI on an unborn baby are not well known. Any woman who is, or may be, pregnant, should carefully discuss this issue with her doctor and radiologist before undergoing a scan.

Types of Results

A normal MRI, MRA, MRS, or MRCP result is one that shows the patient's physical condition to fall within normal ranges for the target area scanned.

Generally, MRI is prescribed only when serious symptoms or negative results from other tests indicate a need. There often exists strong evidence of a condition that the scan is designed to detect and assess. Thus, the results will often be abnormal, confirming the earlier diagnosis. At that point, further testing and appropriate medical treatment is needed. For example, if the MRI indicates the presence of a brain tumor, an MRS may be prescribed to determine the type of tumor so that aggressive treatment can begin immediately without the need for a surgical biospy.

Ultrasound

By Howard Sochurek

Ultrasound has a long and complex history. Some of its earliest uses were military and industrial. Ultrasound was used in primitive submarine navigation systems during World War I. During the 1920s, industrial uses of ultrasound centered on finding flaws in metal sheets or joints. Austrian physician Karl Dussik made the first attempts at medical ultrasound imaging during World War II. After the war, the technology was used mainly for treatment, but by the late 1950s various pioneers developed ways to use it for diagnosis. As a noninvasive, nonradioactive imaging technology, ultrasound has since achieved wide acceptance among both providers and patients. In fact, ultrasound has come to be one of the most widely used imaging techniques. By now many people have had the opportunity to see live-action pictures of their interiors thanks to the ubiquitous technology.

In this selection Howard Sochurek describes how the technology works. A transducer, which operates both as a transmitter and receiver, is placed on the patient's body and then moved across the area under investigation to produce an image. It does this by emitting ultra-high frequency sound waves whose echo from within the body is picked up by the microphone and assembled into an image. Sochurek points to the use of ultrasound to monitor fetal development as one of the technology's greatest boons. The development of Doppler ultrasound has enhanced the value of the technology. Sochurek explains that color Doppler images show subtle variations in movement that can help to evaluate blood flow.

Howard Sochurek is an author and photographer who has produced many illustrated books and articles. The book from which this selection is excerpted first appeared in January 1987 as an article in *National Geographic* magazine.

My earliest remembrance of a doctor is a grandfatherly man in a white coat with a stethoscope dangling from his neck. I remember him gingerly thumping my chest with his fingers while listening carefully. This technique is called percussion, where air or fluid-filled spaces in the body can be detected by a difference in sound when the skin surface is tapped. It has been used by doctors since at least the eighteenth century.

The most modern use of sound in medical diagnosis is sonography or ultrasound (US) imaging, and the images it produces are unique: I saw and heard my own blood flowing through the carotid artery in my neck; watched a human fetus suck its tiny thumb, withdraw it, and give a wide-mouthed, stretching yawn; and watched as a famous neurosurgeon located a brain tumor with a baton-like probe that slowly followed the contours of a shimmering, open brain.

US is one of the simplest and least expensive imaging techniques available to the radiologist today. In clinical use for about 20 years (some of the first US images were produced at the National Institute of Health in 1968), its application has grown exponentially. The original technology for sound imaging came from Defense Department research in underwater sonar dating back to 1942, and even earlier when airborne radar was developed in the 30's. Today [1988], approximately 7,000 hospitals in the United States have US facilities and over 5 million sonography procedures are done each year. Coupled with the computer, many new applications are being devised.

How It Works

To generate a US image a transducer (transmitter-receiver) in the shape of a small rod-like (sometimes flat or square) microphone is placed in contact with the surface of the body. A signal of high frequency in the range of 2 to 10 MHz (millions of cycles per second) is transmitted through the skin. The transducer is passed in an arc over the area of the body being investigated. This arc is repeated line after line, until the full width and depth of the area is covered. A scattering occurs when the pulse hits a dense object within the body. A portion of the pulse is then reflected back to the surface of the skin where the transducer now acts as a receiver (microphone). The time delay between sending the pulse and receiving the reflection determines the depth of the target. The size, shape, texture, and location of the target can also be interpreted by variations in the scatter and reflection signals of the original pulse. A picture is displayed on a computer screen almost immediately as the radiologist or technician makes the line-by-line scan.

One of US's great contributions to diagnostic medicine is in the study of human fetal development, where it has provided a mass of new information. Some doctors feel it will be a basis for the development of fetal medicine as a new subspecialty.

Using Imaging to Estimate Age

Determining the age of the developing fetus using US is now a standard procedure. Beautiful images can be obtained at five weeks when the fetus is just 5 mm long (even its heartbeat can be detected). Calibrated images can also be obtained over a period of time to analyze growth patterns. The size of the skull, abdomen, and femur shaft can be accurately measured. The exact time when a fetus' lungs are capable of breathing independently can be determined. This information is vital to women in premature labor where early delivery would be fatal to the child.

Fetal weight can be determined by volume measurement and is accurate within 50 grams in birth weights from 500 to 4,000 grams. Growth retardation (a near linear increase in growth should occur after ten weeks) often signals problems.

Fetal anatomy can also be studied and abnormalities such as neural tube brain defects and congenital heart problems can be spotted as early as five months.

Discoveries like these have resulted in a whole new field of prenatal and neonatal surgery. Ultrasound-guided procedures such as the administering of medication by injection to the fetus, and drainage of excessive fluids by needle aspiration (withdrawal by suction) have become acceptable and almost routine.

Saving Lives with Ultrasound

One of the stalwarts in US, first at Massachusetts General Hospital in Boston and now at Rush-Presbyterian-St. Luke's Medical Center in Chicago, is Dr. Jason Birnholz. He performed his first US exam at Georgetown University Hospital in Washington, D.C. in 1968. Dr. Birnholz bubbles with excitement over his new discoveries and their latest applications. He explains: "I can see the lacework of fibers, how an organ is structured, or the elasticity of tissue. I can see a firm liver vs. a floppy or water-logged liver. The presence of collagen, a protein found in the ligaments which has unique reflective properties, determines elasticity. The amount of elasticity can be directly related to disease. I can look at fat: fat content is important in diagnosis of liver disease, in cirrhosis, leukemia, and tumors."

Dr. Birnholz told me of a recent case where the use of US saved a life.

A young school teacher in her 30th week of pregnancy came to the hospital for a routine US scan. Dr. Birnholz noticed that the mother's abdomen was much larger than it should have been and that there was excessive fluid around the baby. On the US scan he saw that the baby's mouth was wide open, that the mouth never changed position, and that the tongue was stretched far forward. Close investigation disclosed a large tumor growing in the throat and neck just under the jaw. A fetus actually begins to swallow after 16 weeks, and the tumor was preventing this.

Dr. Birnholz relayed his findings and films to a pediatric surgeon at St. Luke's Hospital, Dr. Lauren Holinger, who stood by with a surgical team as the baby was delivered. At birth the baby turned blue and was near death. It couldn't breathe, the tumor clogging the air passages to the lungs. Immediate action by the surgical team opened the windpipe, and later the tumor was removed.

Today that child, Joseph Ward, is a happy, healthy boy whose life was saved because of the diagnosis achieved through US.

As in Joseph Ward's case, US's great value is that it emits no ionizing radiation and—unlike CT [computer tomography]—can be used on pregnant patients. It images soft tissue densities and discriminates them well, detects tumors and lesions, gallstones and kidney stones, images the flow of blood in the major arteries, and is the modality of choice in examining the prostate gland for a possibility of cancer.

Ultrasound is also routinely used in brain surgery. A portable US unit is taken into the operating room, and after the skull is opened the transducer is placed in contact with the brain to locate the tumor (sound will not pass through bone). . . . Some tumors cannot be seen by even the most experienced neurosurgeons. It is imperative that only diseased tissue be removed, otherwise, brain damage could occur. It is equally important that all of the tumor be removed; if not, the tumor could grow back and repeat surgery would be required. The US scan can provide an accurate view, to a resolution of about one 1 mm, of a tumor's position and size.

A new acquisition of the sonographer is digital color Doppler. Assisted by a computer, Doppler shows in picture and sound the flow and eddying currents of human blood.

The Doppler effect was first explained by Austrian physicist Christian Johann Doppler in 1842, and refers to the change in the frequency of sound as an object moves in distance and velocity from a given point. If you are transmitting soundwaves through a blood vessel, the way the sound is returned can signify subtle changes in blood flow. For example, if the blood is flowing smoothly, the sound will resemble a smoothly flowing brook or stream; if the surface over which the blood flows is irregular, there will be an irregularity in the sound. One use of Doppler is in diagnosing an embolism or occlusion of an artery in a patient who has had a stroke. Irregular pressures and flow patterns result just as if a rock had broken loose and was disrupting the flow of a stream. Doppler allows the radiologist to see and hear how much irregularity exists or whether the blood is flowing at all.

Because US is noninvasive, with little or no discomfort to the patient, I was anxious to see and hear how my own arteries were functioning. I visited Dr. Anthony DeMaria, Chief of Cardiology, at the University of Kentucky Hospital in Lexington, and a proponent of cardiac US.

Seeing the Heart in Action

I removed all my clothing from the waist up and lay back on a semi-reclining bed in a small room. First Dr. DeMaria applied a thick grease-like salve to my skin over the area of my chest (this assures good contact of the transducer to the skin). Earphones were placed on my head so I would hear the action of my heart. Then, taking the transducer in his right hand and making firm contact with the chest, he moved it in short circular arcs over the skin, just below the ribs. Line by line, in color, my throbbing, pulsing heart was displayed on a small monitor. I could both hear and see the butterfly action of my heart valves, see the oxygen-rich blood eddying up through the ventricles, the oxygen-poor blood eddying down, the flecks and pulses of color swirling and whirling through the heart chambers.

Another expert in US imaging, Dr. Steven Horii at NYU Medical Center, has seen the patient load double from 20 patients a day to 40 patients a day in the eight years he has been doing US. His department examines 5,000 patients a year and uses four scanners. Each of the cases is evaluated by either himself or Dr. B. Nagesh Raghavendra, who heads the department. Dr. Horii told me that patients are scheduled about 45 minutes apart, with an average scan time of 30 minutes. A technician handles the procedure with a radiologist doing the scanning in difficult or serious cases, or when the confirmation of a finding is required.

As we talked, Dr. Horii viewed films brought to him by a technician on the completion of the scans. After his evaluation, the patient was released. In one case some indication of a testicular tumor appeared and Horii personally reconfirmed the finding. "You need years of looking at US films to build a mental reference library," commented Dr. Horii. I asked the doctor for cases where his diagnosis had been a life saver and he told me about the case of Mary Masliah.

Pregnancy Gone Wrong

A life-threatening problem in pregnancy exists when the fertilized ovum begins growing outside the uterine cavity. Called an ectopic pregnancy, very few symptoms exist in the initial stages: light vaginal spotting or light bleeding might be the only warning. But the problem is serious since unpredictable hemorrhage can easily occur very suddenly.

Mary came for a routine scan in her tenth week of pregnancy. Her obstetrician was concerned that her uterus was smaller than it should have been and she was experiencing some slight spotting, but no major pain or discomfort.

Dr. Horii found, on viewing the films, the developing embryo clearly visible at the junction of the right fallopian tube and the uterus. Its continued growth threatened the main uterine artery and a major hemorrhage was certainly possible, if not inevitable. This is called a cornual pregnancy and no other imaging technique could have been used to find it without radiation risk. Mary's pregnancy was terminated surgically.

Dr. Horii sees a great and growing future for US. In the past six months [in 1988], he has been using transrectal and transvaginal equipment, in which a transducer is placed on the end of a probe and inserted into the rectum or vagina. In each case, by using a higher frequency signal, greater resolution is obtained. Prostate cancer, so common in elderly men, can be determined by a rectal US probe; the vaginal probe assists in early detection of embryonic abnormalities.

Ultrasound diagnosis was a life saver for little William Mahoney of Manlius, New York. His story was told by Dr. Beverly Spirt, a noted radiologist at SUNY Health Sciences Center in Syracuse, and by Will's mother, Mrs. Catherine Mahoney. Mrs. Mahoney was told of the advent of twins in the eighth week of her pregnancy during a routine US examination. William and his sister Greer were born on January 10, 1983; both were normal.

But at about age two, Willy experienced periodic vomiting attacks that grew increasingly worse. Some lasted as long as ten or twelve hours. Initially diagnosed as a "viral attack," the wretching continued and no medication seemed to work. At wits end, Mrs. Mahoney persisted in getting a second and third opinion. A barium GI series of x-rays disclosed nothing. Heart and head studies were negative and brain tumors and epilepsy were ruled out. The attacks continued, one lasting 14 hours.

In desperation, William's father called his cousin, a cardiologist. He recommended a US scan and Mrs. Mahoney contacted Dr. Spirt in nearby Syracuse. A life-threatening kidney malfunction with a serious duct abnormality was discovered (ureteropelvic junction obstruction or UPJO for short), and surgery was performed the next day. A plastic implant was made to replace the faulty ureter junction, and Willy recovered after eight weeks of convalescence. His surgeon now monitors William's left kidney twice a year with US to observe the implant and confirm that the kidney is functioning normally.

Dr. Spirt told me other stories of patients whose lives have been saved or prolonged by an accurate diagnosis based on US images.

Useful for Kidney Diagnosis

A 32-year-old woman with a newly transplanted kidney was suffering from extreme pain. Ultrasound found four large areas of fluid around the kidney. These buildups are common and result from surgical procedures used in transplant operations. The fluid was removed by needle aspiration and the patient is now fine. Ultrasound is also helpful in evaluating transplanted kidney rejection. Another case involved a fetus with excess fluid in the brain (hydrocephalus) which was properly diagnosed before birth. Immediately after birth, a shunt for drainage of the fluid was implanted; the young lad, now three, is thriving.

Fifty percent of US scans are now performed on obstetrical patients, but as new Doppler ultrasound machines come into general use more and more applications will be in the analysis of heart disease and heart function. Dr. Christopher Merritt at the Ochsner Clinic in New Orleans looks for Doppler to be used in observing the blood flow in all parts of the body. He sees the possibility of early cancer detection. "Cancer induces the formation of new blood vessels which are not normal. We will look at the tissues that are supplied by these blood vessels which may be some of the earliest changes we can perceive."

Revealing Sad News

During our visit, Dr. Merritt proceeded with a routine scan of a young mother in her 28th week of pregnancy. She was thrilled as we watched the fetus kick and turn, suck its thumb, seem to cross its legs, and finally give a huge yawn. Only about half of the parents want to know the sex of their child which can often be determined as early as 15 weeks (males earlier). But, of course, all of them want that first Polaroid snapshot of the TV screen showing the fetus in utero. That psychological process, called bonding, now begins before the child's birth.

With all the joy these few moments held for the child's mother, Dr. Merritt and myself, Dr. Merritt had a much sadder duty to perform that afternoon. As I readied to leave, I found him seated in a small side office consoling a sobbing expectant mother. The US scan had determined that the child she was carrying had died. There was no movement, no heartbeat, no sign of life of any kind, only a silent motionless form on the flickering screen, hands over its head, knees tucked under its chin, asleep forever.

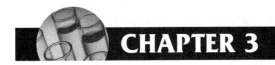

CHAPTER 3

Contemporary Issues in Medical Imaging

Mammography Is Unreliable

By Maryann Napoli

Mammography is an X-ray imaging procedure that allows doctors to search for signs of breast cancer. The health value of mammography has been controversial since 1993, when a Canadian study found no benefit from it for women under the age of fifty, and no additional benefit for women over fifty who had physical examinations of their breasts. In the following selection consumer health advocate Maryann Napoli argues that cancer organizations and companies manufacturing mammography technology have convinced women that mammograms will help them survive breast cancer by detecting it early. In fact, she asserts, the National Cancer Institute (NCI) and the American Cancer Society promoted the procedure long before the evidence of whether it benefits women had accumulated. She writes that there is no evidence that catching breast cancer early results in less drastic treatment. Moreover, mammography produces many false positives that have resulted in some women undergoing unnecessary mastectomies. After the Canadian study, she notes, the NCI withdrew its recommendation that women in their forties get mammograms. Maryann Napoli is associate director of the Center for Medical Consumers in New York City.

My organization, the Center for Medical Consumers, is founded on the belief that people should be encouraged to base their medical treatment decisions on the published evidence. We also believe that screening decisions should be held to the highest standard of evidence because they affect healthy people.

When the National Cancer Institute (NCI) announced its 1993 decision to withdraw the mammography screening recommendation for women in their 40s, I believe that it made the correct judgment. But this didn't seem to change many opinions. Women had already been sold the idea that early detection of breast cancer at any age virtually guarantees cure. The two most common reactions I heard from women at that time were: "I'll still have mammograms just to play it safe" and "What can we do to protect ourselves, if they take away mammography?" To many, it seemed inconceivable that finding a tumor early could be anything but beneficial. At the very least, many women reasoned, finding a breast cancer early would mean a less drastic treatment—a widespread misperception. National breast cancer trials in 1985, for example, found that a lumpectomy and radiation are as effective as mastectomy for women with tumors as large as four centimeters (or even with a tumor that has spread to the lymph nodes).

Facts Get Overlooked

But facts such as this didn't seem to matter. In a scenario I have observed many times, be it a public forum on breast cancer or a radio show, the speaker who points to the lack of scientific evidence to support mammography screening for younger women invariably triggers this response from a member of the audience: "How dare you say that mammography has no benefit to women in their 40s, my breast cancer was discovered on a mammogram last year when I was 43. Now my life has been saved."

The overly optimistic opinions surrounding mammography screening's value to women in their 40s are the direct result of promoting a technology to the public before there was clear scientific evidence proving benefit. In the early 1970s, before there was any scientific evidence to prove mammography's benefit to younger women, the American Cancer Society (ACS) and the NCI began to promote screening for all women over the age of 35. The message to the public was—and still is—"breast cancer is curable, if detected early enough." What was merely a hunch on the part of ACS and NCI was presented to the public as established truth.

While a woman's doctor may be the most influential factor in determining whether she will undergo mammography screening, the most influential source of information for the lore surrounding mammography screening—for the overly optimistic expectations surrounding mammography—is the ACS. The ACS has a long history of overstating the case for early detection, of using five-year survival statistics to imply cure, of recommending screening tests before there is scientific evidence to prove safety and efficacy, and of not warning of mammography's downside, specifically the uncertainties surrounding ductal carcinoma in situ (DCIS).

Misdiagnosis Leads to Mastectomy

In 1977 the public learned about these so-called "microscopic cancers" that caused 64 women to be misdiagnosed as having breast cancer in one set of trials; 37 had undergone mastectomy. Quite a revelation. No one ever warns the public about finding a cancer so early that pathologists aren't sure that it's cancer. And here we are 20 years later, and pathologists are still trying to determine the natural history of the different subtypes of DCIS in order to avoid overtreatment.

Now, there's a new generation of women in their 40s who were too young at the time of those 1977 headlines to be concerned about mammography-related misdiagnoses. After all, breast cancer in that era was an older woman's disease. Women now in their 40s have been "raised" on the public health message that "breast cancer is curable if found early enough." In other words, cure is simply a matter of finding breast cancer early.

Yet in 1980, I would come across a review of all published breast cancer trials in the *New England Journal of Medicine* which found that 25%–35% of all women diagnosed and treated at Stage I developed metastasis anyway and died within ten years of their mastectomies. This is just one of many contradictions I would find between the "public education" message to women and the published evidence.

In 1985, we saw the start of breast cancer awareness activities, initiated and largely sponsored by Zeneca, the manufacturer of tamoxifen, a cancer treatment. Now it is the corporate ads like those of DuPont and General Electric (GE), makers of mammography-related equipment, that feature the same old misleading statistics. A recent GE ad for breast cancer awareness month, for example, claimed "a remarkable 91% cure rate" for its new, improved mammography equipment. What does this mean? The figure refers to the proportion of women who now live for at least five years after diagnoses and treatment—not an accurate measure of cure.

These corporate ads come cloaked in the aura of public service announcements (PSAs). And frankly, in terms of half-truths, I don't find them to be any different than the real PSAs sponsored by the ACS or the American College of Radiology. The depiction of young women in these ads, the use of misleading "one in eight" and "one in nine" statistics, which refer to risk over a lifetime, not during a woman's 40s, and the magazines and talk shows featuring personal stories of young breast cancer survivors have all contributed to the impression of breast cancer as a young woman's disease. Put this heightened awareness together with the exaggerated "public health message"—early detection equals cure—and you have a lot of women out there who think that a mammogram is the only thing that stands between them and imminent death from breast cancer.

Mammography proponents invariably frame the debate in this manner: what's the harm of anxiety over an abnormal mammogram or a biopsy compared to death from breast cancer? Well, we don't know whether any deaths are prevented, and many women (including those over age 50) do not fully understand the third possibility associated with mammography screening: misdiagnosis of cancer—the over-reading of atypical benign breast disease as carcinoma in situ, or of in situ disease as invasive cancer. Such diagnostic errors have occurred in several major trials where pathologists would be expected to be more expert than those in the real world. I have met many a woman who has had a mastectomy for DCIS, who regards herself as a cancer survivor, who worries about recurrence like every other cancer patient, who believes her daughters are at high risk, and who has no idea of the uncertainties that surround her diagnosis or that evidence suggests that only some cases of DCIS will become invasive cancer.

Most women today with a diagnosis of DCIS come to our center knowing something about the controversies surrounding it. But the point is they hear it for the first time at diagnosis, not before they consent to screening in the first place.

Traditionally, cancer survivors become evangelists for screening, but I've detected less enthusiasm of late. Every breast cancer activist I know is a woman diagnosed in her 40s. These women know firsthand about mammography's other problem: its high false-negative rate for younger women.

False Positives

Women who have a mammogram every year during their 40s run a 30% chance of being told that the X-ray shows an abnormality, even though their breasts are normal. The vast majority of these women then will have unnecessary biopsies, some even mastectomies.

New evidence from Sweden shows a 24% reduction in breast cancer mortality. For nearly a year, radiologists have been portraying this finding to the public as the proof that now ends the controversy. But what, for example, does the reduction in "subsequent" mortality actually mean? (The public never hears that qualifying word.) Is this finding an argument for starting screening at age 40, or for delaying it until age 50? How does a woman weigh the 24% reduction in subsequent mortality against her odds of misdiagnosis? Does this mean that everyone who undergoes mammography screening can reduce her personal odds of dying of breast cancer by 24% (which is how most people interpret such a statistic)?

Perhaps it is fairer to put it this way: Mammography screening will result in a prolonged life for 24% of women with breast cancers. The majority of women whose cancers are found on a mammogram, however, will be unaffected by early detection, either because they have an aggressive, fast-growing cancer or because the tumor is so slow-growing, the women would enjoy long-term survival whether it was found early on a mammogram or later, once a symptom appeared. Some women will be falsely assured that they are cancer-free.

I have contacted several advocacy organizations and heard variations on this theme: "We'll continue to have mammograms, but researchers must find better ways to detect early breast cancers because mammography does not help most women. We need to know more about what causes breast cancer." Mammography may be the best detection tool we have, as the PSAs constantly remind women, but it's just not good enough.

The recent Consensus Panel, by educating women and their doctors about what mammography can and cannot do, may bring to the topic a large dose of reality.

Mammography Is Reliable

By Amy Langer, interviewed by Erica Heilman

Despite some studies suggesting that mammography—the X-raying of breasts—provides no health benefit, the procedure still has many advocates. In the selection that follows health and medicine journalist Erica Heilman interviews one such advocate. Amy Langer, representing an alliance of breast cancer organizations, argues that mammograms can detect cancers at an early stage, which makes it easier to cure the patient. A woman whose breast cancer is caught by mammography before it is large enough to be detected by manual exam has, Langer claims, a better than 90 percent chance of being successfully treated. Langer asserts that there is a consensus among government and private organizations that women over forty should have yearly mammograms. Amy Langer is the executive director of the National Alliance of Breast Cancer Organizations.

For years, the National Cancer Institute and the American Cancer Society have recommended that women over forty receive regular mammograms so that tumors may be detected in their earlier, more treatable stages.

But these recommendations have come under the sharp scrutiny of two Danish researchers who say that the current standards are "unjustified". Their findings, published in the British medical journal the *Lancet*, were critical of methods used in several large screening trials in the U.K., North America and Sweden. Since then even more data has come out on both sides.

What is a woman to think?

Below, Amy Langer, Executive Director of the National Alliance of Breast Cancer Organizations, explains why many international public health and breast cancer experts have dismissed the *Lancet* findings, and continue to strongly recommend regular mammograms for women forty and older.

Erica Heilman: To begin, what is the National Alliance of Breast Cancer Organizations, or NABCO?

Amy Langer: NABCO is a 16-year-old non-profit organization that is the nation's leading information and education resource about breast cancer.

Why Screening Is Important

Heilman: Could you first describe why breast cancer screening is important?

Langer: Breast cancer is the most common form of cancer in women in the United States. Women have a one in nine chance of being diagnosed in their lifetimes, and particularly at age 50, the risk starts climbing.

Mammograms find breast cancers at small sizes, before they can even be felt by women and their doctors. The smaller the size of a breast cancer found, the easier it is to treat it successfully.

In the vast majority of cases, breast cancer detected early is treated without losing the breast, and with drug therapy that reduces the chances that breast cancer will return. When breast cancer is detected by a mammogram—when too small to be felt—the chance for successful treatment is extremely high—over 90 percent. In fact, breast cancers these days are being reported at about half the size they were as recently as a decade ago.

Heilman: And what are the current breast cancer screening recommendations?

Langer: The national consensus screening recommendation—which is an opinion of the National Cancer Institute, every major government agency, the American Cancer Society, the American Medical Association and literally dozens of other leading medical and women's health organizations—is that women should have regular screening mammograms—that is, before any signs or symptoms of breast cancer—starting at age forty.

Heilman: What is the controversy about?

Langer: What's going on right now is an extension of confusion that all of us had hoped was resolved, and is effectively an academic controversy over methodology. There's been some disagreement about maturing results of worldwide breast cancer screening studies.

The data that the Danish team is discussing and reanalyzing are from studies around the world that have been completed for a long time. Most of them started over thirty years ago.

All the trials were a little different in design. Methodology did differ from trial to trial somewhat, and some of the screening methods were different. They were similar enough, however, so that it was statistically appropriate to pool their results.

The data that came out of these trials was sufficiently compelling to convince all of the leading academic, government and professional organizations that regular mammograms were an appropriate and beneficial public-health recommendation for women in the United States. And women listened and started getting them.

Heilman: What has happened as a result of these recommendations?

Langer: Recent studies over the last couple years indicate that up to three-quarters of age-eligible insured women are getting mammograms. And the mammograms are finding breast cancers at an earlier stage and at smaller sizes.

The Studies

Heilman: So which are the studies that women need to be most concerned with?

Langer: What's more important than what happened in a 1972 study is what's going on in the clinic every day. We have recent studies from major cancer centers and data in our national cancer databases that show what's known as a 'downward stage shift', or the diminishing, earlier stage at which breast cancer is being diagnosed.

In the real world, breast cancers are getting smaller, and that means not only are they easier to treat and increasingly survivable, but there are far more treatment options for women managing their disease.

Heilman: But some argue that mammograms can lead to treatment of tumors that may not pose a threat to a woman's life. Is over-treatment a problem?

Langer: The way I usually answer that question is to say yes and no. When you look at the breast, you find a lot of things. Among the things that we find with screening mammography are very early, preinvasive breast cancers—most commonly ductal carcinoma in situ (DCIS). And we don't know enough about the natural history of preinvasive breast cancers to know which we can leave alone and which need to be removed . . . the kind of breast cancer that can travel and kill. This can put women and their doctors in the difficult position of not understanding what is best to do.

On the flip side, for breast cancers that we do know for certain are life-threatening, we're finding them earlier and treating the disease more successfully.

Heilman: So the answer lies in thorough education about preinvasive cancer during the screening process?

Langer: Education is essential. But to some extent, I think that you can get lost in what's really important if you allow yourself to get bogged down with presenting a woman with every nuance of how preinvasive breast cancer could behave. Women are mostly interested in, "What's important for me? What makes sense for me? And what should I do?"

I think it is important for women to realize that if they have breast cancer, finding it early is still the best bet for successful treatment. If along the way there are some quandaries, extra biopsies, or suspicious lesions and preinvasive disease, well, that is the price that is paid. But I think it is a price worth paying.

Relying on Experts

Heilman: Why must a governing body make these recommendations? Why shouldn't a woman decide alone with her doctor whether to get screened, and when?

Langer: Because we cannot be experts in everything. As women who juggle and multitask constantly, we need to rely on someone to be a resident expert. And that someone should be the most qualified body and group that has reviewed data, understands health tradeoffs, has a high degree of ethical responsibility and is made up of experts committed to patient empowerment through providing all approximate information.

You can't find that in one body anywhere. So one of the things that I think is most convincing about screening mammography as an issue, is that an extremely diverse group of expert organizations have either recommended—if that's their business, like the American Cancer Society or the NCI—or have supported—like NABCO and other nonprofits have done—ongoing screening, for women forty and older, with regular mammograms.

Heilman: What do you suggest to women who are confused by this recent controversy?

Langer: I don't think that this debate needs to turn women into researchers or scientists or academic police. I think we need to rely on experts. And, of course, discuss the issue with our own doctors.

But I'm not shy, and as a well-known voice for women's astonishing, often under-represented ability to make decisions about their own health, this is not one I think should be left to flipping a coin. The data is here, it's solid. Until someone can show us something new or prove otherwise, we are all comfortable that mammography—regular screening mammography—makes sense.

That's Me All Over

By Alan Farnham

For those who worry about their health, the opportunity to get a peek inside their own bodies may be irresistible. Beginning in the late 1990s, the marketplace responded by offering consumers what are generally known as "whole body scans," which are detailed computed tomography scans from the neck to the torso. In the following selection Alan Farnham describes his experience undergoing the procedure, which he terms a full body scan. As Farnham explains, he opted to undergo a "virtual colonoscopy" at the same time. This involves inflating the colon so that the CT scan image its interior while making its pass around the patient's body. Farnham lauds the virtual colonoscopy as an alternative to the "invasive and messy" procedure of inserting a fiber optic tube into the colon to check for possibly cancerous growths known as polyps. He also appreciates the comprehensive nature of the full body scan. In addition to looking for polyps, he writes, the scan can identify nodules in the lungs or plaque in the arteries. Although the whole body scan cannot find every lurking hazard, and although medical insurers will not pay for it, Farnham argues that the procedure is worth its cost because it provides peace of mind. Alan Farnham writes on lifestyle issues for *Forbes* magazine.

New body-scanning technology promises to capture incipient diseases in glorious 3-D, without the dreaded prod. You'll never look at yourself the same way again.

Lying on a cool, vinyl-padded bed in a doctor's office in Manhattan, I brace myself for one of the hottest new procedures in modern medicine. First step: an entirely different kind of inflation. "Now, go easy," the nurse says as she hands over a rubber bulb attached to a long tube inserted, ahem, right up into my backside.

It is time to pump myself up. Gradually, resting now and then, I squeeze the bulb 50 times to fill my body with air. Soon I begin to feel like the Michelin man, bloated but not especially uncom-

Alan Farnham, "That's Me All Over," *Forbes*, vol. 168, October 29, 2001, p. 230. Copyright © 2001 by Forbes, Inc. Reproduced by permission.

fortable. Comfort—as in peace of mind—was what I was after. The self-inflation was a prerequisite to a "virtual colonoscopy" and an accompanying full-body scan.

Finding Hidden Dangers

This costly but increasingly popular diagnostic technique moves a patient head to toe through a large, cylindrical imaging machine in less than 30 minutes. The startling images that result from this "fantastic voyage," sans Raquel Welch, will let doctors pinpoint the hidden flaws that may kill me—polyps in the colon, plaque in the arteries, malignant nodules in the lungs from that one cigarette I smoke every day.

Body scans are far less invasive and messy than poking a periscope into your innards, and they are more comprehensive than getting a stress test or having one organ checked at a time with, say, X rays or ultrasound. The new machines, using a technology called electron beam tomography, shoot images up to ten times as fast as an older CT (computerized tomography) scan, able to capture an intricate picture of the heart in between beats. The new technique can spot lung nodules that are only one-fifth the size of what can be found by an X ray. "It's like putting the chest through a bread slicer," says Dr. Geoffrey Bodeau, codirector of the HeartScan Minnesota clinic in Minneapolis. Data captured by the scanner are manipulated by software to create 3-D images of interior anatomy. At some clinics, doctors guide patients on a visual journey through the twists and turns of their own arteries and plumbing. The results can prod you to change your life.

That happened to Robert Rizzi, a 64-year-old executive who visited my doctor, Allan Rubenstein of New York–based University HeartScan. Rizzi was overweight and had a family history of heart disease. Sure enough, the scan found calcium deposits in three arteries. Says Dr. Rubenstein: "He had to have immediate surgery or undertake a lifestyle change. "Rizzi chose the latter, shedding 28 pounds in two months.

The procedure's rising popularity has brought out the showman in some clinicians. At HealthScreen America, a storefront in Jacksonville, Fla., window-shopping hypochondriacs are lured in by a 4-foot-tall red and blue fiberglass heart, with an artificial brook burbling behind it. A menu lists scan prices at $20 to $1,000, with package deals available.

A Complement to Other Procedures

Scanning has its drawbacks. Dr. Kenneth Cooper of the Cooper Clinic in Dallas has done 35,000 scans since 1997 but says even the latest gear can't spot soft, precalcified plaque that poses a risk of clogging an artery. He says patients also should take a standard stress test to help detect soft blockages.

Cooper won't yet offer the latest wrinkle, virtual colonoscopies, because he says the procedure still isn't good enough to isolate polyps from other matter. A June study in *Radiology* showed that virtual colonoscopies had a 38% rate of false positives, or indications of polyps that didn't exist. And if a virtual tour turns up a real polyp, you'll have to get scoped anyway.

But as a salve for my anxiety, which may be understandable for a 46-year-old who smokes a little, eats a lot and exercises somewhat regularly, the full-body voyage was worth the $1,400 price of admission. (As an elective procedure, insurers rarely cover it, but your odds may improve if you're referred.)

Dr. Rubenstein's office is designed for the busy executive who wants to get in and out in under an hour. After a quick consult, I donned a surgical gown, entered the scanning room and lay down on the pallet. Once inside the large scanner, rubber bulb in hand, I heeded the technicians' voices coming through a speaker, telling me to give more squeezes.

The novelty of self-inflation was distracting enough to ease the anxiety of moving through a giant, humming aperture, with a bright red light at its apex. After a series of four smooth passes—some of which required me to hold my breath for what seemed like a minute—it was over. When the tube was removed, I did not, balloon-like, whiz around the room and bounce off the ceiling.

Clean Bill of Health

Some of the results were available immediately, including a graphic printout ranking my arterial plaque buildup against my age group. The other results were farmed out to local specialists. In less than a week my results were complete: no colon polyps and no heart disease—only a small scar in my left lung (possibly a relic from childhood bronchitis). "Keep doing what you're doing," Dr. Rubenstein advised.

One parting word of advice for those who undergo the virtual colonoscopy: Ten or 15 minutes after it ends, the accumulated air escape. When that happens, you want to make sure you're in a private place—private and maybe soundproof.

Not only does scanning save you the indignity of being plumbed, but the results (depending on the ailment) may not be obtainable by traditional means.

Body Scans Are Not Worth the Risk

By Life Extension Magazine

Computed tomography (CT), the technique of combining multiple X-ray images taken from different angles, can be used to provide a scan of all the vital organs in a single sweep. In the late 1990s entrepreneurs began to market this technique as a "whole body scan," intended to reveal hidden diseases. In the selection that follows, *Life Extension Magazine* explains why whole body scans are risky. The central problem, it says, is unnecessary and hazardous exposure to radiation. A single CT scan of the chest is equivalent to hundreds of conventional X-rays. The direct marketing of full body scans to consumers has raised concerns about excessive radiation exposure within the U.S. Food and Drug Administration and the radiologist community. Moreover, the magazine argues that standard examinations for each of the major organs are more effective and, in some cases, nonradioactive. *Life Extension Magazine* urges readers to weigh the risk of radiation exposure against the supposed peace of mind that a full body scan may provide. The magazine is a publication of the Life Extension Foundation, a nonprofit organization whose goal is to extend the time in which people can live in health, youth, and vigor.

Editor's Note: Since the publication of this and other articles critical of the nonmedical use of CT scans, the New York Times *has reported a collapse in consumer demand for whole body scans.*

Scan centers make body scans sound like they're as safe as a stroll down Fifth Avenue. Our investigation into the scan industry raises grave doubts about the safety of so-called health scans.

Ever considered relaxing in a radioactive bath? Back in the 1920s, you could buy radioactive bath salts. They were a cure for insomnia. Once in bed, you could apply your Radium Ore Healing Pad—a nifty device said to be good for stomach, liver and spine. You might think this is laughable—you wouldn't consider taking a radioactive bath or curling up with a radioactive heating pad. But you might consider getting a body scan—something that may turn out to be just as laughable and far more dangerous in the long run.

Body scans are the latest health fad. A blizzard of media attention has healthy people flocking to "scan centers" to get their bodies scanned. The concept is terrific. State-of-the-art machines known as CTs (computed tomography) "slice" internal organs into wafer-thin serial images that are then viewed on a computer screen. CT scans can reveal cancer, heart disease, osteoporosis and more at their earliest stages. They don't hurt, they're fast and if you've got $700 to $1300, you too can see your insides.

Radiation Hazard

Sounds great and it is great—except for one thing. Radiation. And lots of it. In effective doses, one CT chest scan is the equivalent of 400 chest x rays or 3.6 years of background radiation; a scan of the abdomen 500 chest x rays or 4.5 years of natural background radiation. A scan of the head is the equivalent of 115 chest x rays, or one year of natural background radiation. Combine the chest and abdomen, and you've got a body scan—almost 1,000 x rays (imagine sitting on an x ray table while 1,000 x rays are taken). These are "effective doses", meaning that depending on your body type and the scanner, you could get even more radiation. It's estimated that the risk of a chest x ray causing fatal cancer is 1-in-1,000,000. A CT scan of the abdomen has been estimated to up the risk to 1-in-2,000. All of this for what experienced radiologists say are "unnecessary evaluations".

According to Dr. Robert Stanley, president of the American Roentgen Ray Society, a 45-year-old healthy person who gets one scan doesn't have to worry. But the FDA's Dr. Thomas Shope has cautioned that multiple scans can expose a person to radiation approaching the lower levels of Hiroshima and Nagasaki. A controversial new report estimates that if 600,000 children get head and abdomen CT scans, 500 will get cancer from those scans. The body doesn't forget radiation: it keeps count of every x ray you get. It's important to think about your own lifetime exposure before you volunteer to be irradiated. Radiation damage to DNA is never completely repaired.

So-called "health scans" or "body scans" have gotten the FDA's attention. CT scanners were never intended to be used in people with no symptoms and unknown risk. There are many diagnostics that can be done for a person who is concerned about their health that either don't involve radiation, or involve significantly less. These modalities can be used before a CT scan. CTs were designed as serious diagnostic devices, not health enhancers.

Experienced radiologists are also distancing themselves from whole body scans in a big way. The American Roentgen Ray Society wouldn't be the first place you'd look for a CT critic. Yet its president is highly critical of whole body CT screening in asymptomatic people. Stanley, who knows CTs inside and out, points out that the damage from a body scan might not be evident for many years. CT scans, he says, are much more complex than simply putting a person in a scanner and reading a computer print-out. That's like taking a jet fighter out for a joy ride.

It has been repeatedly proven that CT scans are subjecting people to unnecessarily high levels of radiation. New calls by radiologists themselves for radiation reductions are only the latest in a decades-old demand for radiation reductions. Radiation reductions of 50% or more are possible today without any effect on picture quality. A study published in 1991 on CT scans of the head is typical: "While computed tomography (CT) has become an important imaging modality in the evaluation of the paranasal sinuses, the radiation dose remains higher than is necessary . . . images were of diagnostic quality even when dose levels were reduced by a factor of 28."

Yet despite these kinds of findings, radiologists continue to ignore the issue of radiation exposure, and manufacturers carry on business as usual. The public has been in the dark about radiation and CT scans until recently when the media picked up on studies published in the *American Journal of Roentgenology* showing that CT radiation is off the map. One of the editorials is unprecedented in demanding that CT manufacturers lower the radiation. Another asserts that radiologists have been unaware of or indifferent to the high doses of radiation associated with CTs.

Unregulated Doses

Some scan centers offer "rapid scans"—usually for detecting calcium in arteries. A common perception is that a speedy scan exposes you to less radiation. This isn't necessarily true. "Rapid" scans are like a stop-action camera. They enable radiologists to capture an image of a beating heart or a scanee who moves. In order to do this, the machine must generate more intense radiation. However, although the person undergoing the scan is subjected to more radiation, it is for less time. For this reason, rapid scans expose a scanee to about the same amount of radiation as a regular scan, although some scanners generate more or less than others.

The amount of radiation a scanner generates is not regulated by the FDA [Food and Drug Administration]; however, the agency does require that scan manufacturers disclose the radiation dose to anyone who asks. Excessive radiation exposure is often the end result of the quest for good picture quality. Picture quality is a big selling point for manufacturers. Their promotional material is full of information about how good the pictures are, but virtually silent when it comes to radiation doses.

The next generation of scanners is supposed to automatically adjust the amount of radiation according to a person's own absorption potential. For example, if a child is given the same amount of radiation as an adult, they will be much more affected by it. Similarly, a heavy person will diffuse or divert more of the radiation away from internal organs than a thin person, and be damaged less. The need for automatic adjustment is obvious, yet self-adjusting scanners are not on the market yet.

Alternatives to Heart Scans

Scan centers are offering scans of the heart to detect calcium deposits in coronary arteries. The American Heart Association in collaboration with the American College of Cardiology has issued a statement of non-support of electron-beam computed tomography (EBCT)—rapid scans—for heart disease detection in asymptomatic people. Their position is that rapid scans are no more predictive than usual risk factors. For example, ankle-brachial pressure index—a simple measurement—is highly predictive of whether or not a person with no symptoms will have a heart attack, whether they will die of that heart attack and whether they have narrowing of the arteries. The accuracy of ankle-brachial pressure as an indicator of heart disease risk is on par with smoking, the most predictive indicator. It and homocysteine levels are better predictors of heart disease than cholesterol levels, with one study suggesting that homocysteine is better at predicting the extent of atherosclerosis in low-risk patients than high-risk. C-reactive protein is another predictor. All are simple tests that can be performed at any doctor's office without exposing you to radiation.

The AHA and ACC also point out that CT scans only measure calcium, and calcium is only one facet of heart disease. EBCT does not detect "soft" lesions or unstable plaques. And while the presence of calcium is highly predictive of having a heart attack, the groups argue that false-positives "can result in additional expensive and unnecessary testing to rule out a diagnosis of CAD (coronary artery disease)." In other words, if you get a scan at a scan center and something shows up, you will have to undergo additional tests that may involve more radiation to find out what it means. One of those tests may be the same scan, only this time with intravenous contrast which can illuminate lesions, plaque and the like.

The failure to use intravenous contrast is one of the problems with scan centers. CT scans done at such centers are one-half of a proper scan. The other half is the contrast material. It's the contrast material that tells the story. It enables the radiologist to differentiate between cancer and a benign growth, heart disease and calcification only.

Scans Miss Some Cancers

Another popular scan these days is a CT scan of the gut. "Virtual colonoscopies" appear to have widespread support, with some predicting they will become the next mammogram if they can be improved. However, radiation exposure is one of the hurdles that has to be overcome before virtual colonoscopies replace colonoscopies as the diagnostic tool for colon cancer, according to Dr. Joseph T. Ferrucci of the American Roentgen Ray Society. There are other problems as well.

Colon cancer is the second most deadly cancer in the U.S. (after lung cancer). The number of people who have colon cancer without knowing it is alarming. A study published in the *New England Journal of Medicine* found that 37% of men tested (only some of which were at high risk) had adenomas or invasive cancer without knowing it. Sigmoidoscopy, a procedure where the doctor examines the lowest part of the colon, is inadequate to diagnose this disease. Anyone age 50 or over with average risk factors is advised to get a colonoscopy which can enable the physician to see the entire colon. Men are especially at risk for colon cancer. The good news is that colon cancer responds to treatment if caught early. It's clear that colonoscopies save lives. Unfortunately, the unpleasantness of the procedure keeps some people away until they have symptoms so obvious, they can't ignore them anymore, and by then cancer can be advanced.

Virtual colonoscopy will change all that once it's perfected and put into widespread use. The studies already look very promising on virtual colonoscopy. But there are problems that have to be overcome before virtual colonoscopy replaces traditional colonoscopy. One of them is that although virtual colonoscopy detects most cancers and growths 10 mm or larger, it has trouble with small polyps and flat adenomas. Some cancers are simply undetectable by virtual colonoscopy at this time.

But, unlike other scan procedures where the risks of unnecessary radiation exposure and side effects may outweigh the benefits, the high incidence of colon cancer and the favorable response it has to early detection make the risk/benefit ratio of this CT scan very favorable. Older men are particularly at risk and they should undergo a colonoscopy no matter what. A virtual colonoscopy is better than no colonoscopy, but traditional colonoscopy remains the gold standard for diagnosing colon cancer and precancerous conditions. Young people with no symptoms and no risk factors should not get virtual colonoscopies. If such a person can't sleep at night wondering if they have colon cancer, they should get the traditional colonoscopy that involves no radiation.

Scans Can't Replace Mammograms

As a screening device for breast cancer, CT scans do not work. Some radiologists are alarmed that women might think a chest or body scan can replace a mammogram. There are many differences between a CT scan and a mammogram. Mammograms were designed specifically for screening the breasts. They have a history of development and refinement behind them. They use far less radiation (200 millirads, or approximately eight chest x rays), and they reveal far more. While CT scans can be used for guiding breast biopsies, they are not a good screening device for breast cancer.

Unlike CT scan centers which are regulated by the state only, mammogram facilities have to be certified by the FDA. They must use the lowest radiation possible and they must retain radiologists who read at least 480 mammograms a year and attend continuing education classes. Radiologists who read mammograms have a lot of experience in looking for breast cancer.

Most people don't think about what will happen after the scan. But according to a *Wall Street Journal* report, one scan center sends 80% of its scanees to specialists post-scan. Either a whole lot of people are very sick or scan centers really don't know what they're doing. Stanley points to comments like one recently attributed to the director of a scan center who said that he's never seen a normal body scan—to argue that something is wrong with what they're doing. "Their motivation is misdirected," he argues. CT scans, he says, were never intended to be used without contrast material in asymptomatic people. Scans used in this way can reveal all sorts of "abnormalities". "When you're looking for abnormalities millimeter-by-millimeter, you're going to find them," he says. A person may go through thousands of dollars of unnecessary and invasive tests after a scan, including more radiation, to find out they have . . . nothing. It's like believing every mole on your body is melanoma. Stanley points out that if you take anyone who has died and section their kidneys millimeter-by-millimeter, in 22% of them you will find renal tumors. (A similar situation exists in the liver where "cavernous angiomas" develop.) But these tumors are rarely cancerous, and rarely develop into full-blown cancer which is detectable anyway by other means, is uncommon, and treatable.

Stanley is not against screening. Mammograms and other screening modalities save lives (although he's quick to point out that diagnosing cancer early does not always lower the mortality rate—it depends on the type of cancer). But he and other radiologists are adamantly against asymptomatic people undergoing whole body scans as part of a health program.

Sizing Up the Risks

Let's face it: blanketing yourself with radiation is not healthy. Because there is a risk involved, serious consideration should be given to whether the benefit is likely to be offset by the damage a CT scan does to the body. By all means, a person at risk for a disease, either because of lifestyle or genetics, should get whatever tests they need to assure them they are healthy. In most cases, tests not involving radiation can be done first. These tests should be exhausted before a CT is considered. If a CT scan is warranted, it should be done—correctly, with proper contrast material, by an experienced radiologist in that field. Contrast material increases the ability of the radiologist to detect small cancers, precancerous conditions, and distinguish between something important and something that isn't. If a body scan is chosen as the first-line diagnostic tool and it finds something, chances are the scan will have to be repeated with intravenous contrast material, subjecting the scanee to a double dose of radiation.

Many people who have undergone body scans did so because they weren't doing what they were supposed to do healthwise. The scan motivated them to pay attention to their health. And that would be fine if CT scans were totally benign. They're not, and any person contemplating a scan should ask themselves before they walk into a scan center if they really need a big dose of radiation to provoke them into doing what they already know they should be doing. Ask yourself: do I really need to undergo the equivalent of 1,000 x rays to find out I'm not exercising, I'm not eating right, and I need to buy a better mattress for my aching back? Can motivation and peace-of-mind be obtained another way?

CT scans have a place in diagnostics. To a person with symptoms of a serious disease or serious risk factors (such as smoking or familial heart disease), the benefit of getting a proper scan, with intravenous contrast, outweighs the risk. But the risk/benefit ratio collapses when the person getting a scan is a healthy individual with no symptoms; vague risk factors, and the scan is delivering a whopping dose of radiation. A person truly concerned about their health won't place that bet. We can't feel it, we don't see it, but we've got to believe that radiation is not healthy. We've got to listen to decades of data that tells us that radiation is something to be avoided when possible. Otherwise, we might as well sleep with Radium Ore Healing Pads tucked under our pillows, as the manufacturer of those devices once suggested.

Screening for Lung Cancer May Do More Harm than Good

By Liz Szabo

Medical imaging has proven useful in detecting numerous forms of cancer. In this selection, however, reporter Liz Szabo explains that doctors have yet to find a reliable imaging method to detect lung cancer in time to save the life of the patient. About three-quarters of those with lung cancer die, despite detection of their lesions by X-ray. The most promising advance to date, she reports, has been spiral computed tomography (CT) scans. Some doctors have begun advising patients who are smokers to have annual CT checkups. However, no proof exists that these scans help, whereas risks are known to exist. The big questions are whether the advanced technology actually can catch lung cancer at an earlier stage, and if so, whether that will help the patient survive it. Some preliminary studies suggest that CT lung screenings can help save lives. However, some experts remain skeptical. They note that false positives are common events in such screenings, and that follow-up procedures can be painful and even dangerous. Liz Szabo reports on medical and health issues for *USA Today*.

Doctors can screen for cancers of the cervix, prostate, breast and colon.

But they have no reliable way to test for a disease that kills more people than those malignancies combined: lung cancer.

Doctors have tried a number of procedures, such as chest

X-rays, but have been disappointed that no test has been proved to save lives. The most promising lung cancer screening method so far seems to be spiral computed tomography, or CT scans, which provide 3D images of the lungs.

Some doctors recommend annual spiral CT scans for heavy smokers. A growing number of medical centers aggressively market lung scans, which are generally not covered by insurance, to nervous smokers and ex-smokers willing to pay hundreds of dollars out-of-pocket.

Many scientists, however, note that there is no clear proof that spiral CT scans prevent death. With no proven benefits—but real risks—lung screenings could do more harm than good, critics say. In particular, many experts worry that imprecise results could lead to additional tests that are unnecessary and even dangerous.

Putting It to the Test

To test the technology, the National Cancer Institute has launched the $ 200 million National Lung Screening Trial. With 50,000 patients at 34 medical centers, it's the largest lung cancer screening study ever.

"It's one of the most important cancer prevention studies in the world," says Edward Gelmann, a professor of oncology and medicine at Georgetown's Lombardi Comprehensive Cancer Center in Washington. "If it doesn't work, it will save everybody a lot of money," says Gelmann, Georgetown's lead researcher for the study. "If it works, it has the opportunity to save a lot of lives."

Americans spend more than $ 5 billion a year to take care of people with lung cancer, the leading cause of cancer death that claims 157,200 Americans a year.

Doctors say the trial will answer important questions about CT scans.

"What we don't know is: Will these tests really find lung cancer early?" says Len Lichtenfeld, deputy chief medical officer for the American Cancer Society. "Does finding it early make a difference? What else does it find? And does it harm the patient when you find it early?"

The study is designed as a "randomized controlled trial."

All patients are smokers or ex-smokers, who account for 87% of lung cancer patients. Doctors will follow patients for about seven years, comparing death rates of patients randomly assigned to undergo CT scans with those receiving chest X-rays.

Some experts say the trial would be more effective if it included a third group of unscreened patients. NCI officials noted that they considered adding an unscreened group, which would have required enrolling an additional 25,000 participants and greatly increased the costs.

Scientists have searched for a dependable lung cancer screening method for four decades.

Early Detection Saves Lives

When tumors are caught in the earliest stage, 70% of patients survive, according to the U.S. Preventive Services Task Force, an influential panel of experts that evaluates screening methods. But only 5% of patients survive after being diagnosed with the most advanced kind of tumor.

By the time that patients are diagnosed with lung cancer today, 75% have incurable tumors.

Doctors first screened for cancer in the 1950s and 1960s, using chest X-rays and samples of sputum coughed up from the lung, Lichtenfeld says. Large studies performed since the 1970s, however, found that although those methods detected some cancers, they missed many others and did not reduce mortality. In six studies, scientists found no benefit to either X-rays or sputum tests.

Like X-rays, spiral CT scans—a newer technology—are quick and painless. Both expose patients to radiation. But studies show that CT scans detect about six times as many early lung cancers than X-rays, says Claudia Henschke, a radiology professor at Weill Medical College of Cornell University.

Spiral CT scans can spot tumors that are about 1 centimeter wide. X-rays typically pick up tumors that are 2 centimeters or larger, Henschke says.

In an influential 1999 study, Henschke and her colleagues found that CT scans detected lung cancers earlier than X-rays did.

Since then, Henschke and researchers from 36 institutions have screened 27,000 people with CT scans and have found 400 patients with cancer. Preliminary results show that only 16 of those patients have died from lung cancer since 1993. Her results have not yet been published.

Some experts, however, wonder whether CT scans are too sensitive.

False Alarms

In Henschke's studies, initial scans find suspicious lung lesions in up to 15% of patients, very few of whom actually have cancer. Other studies of CT scans have found "abnormalities" in up to 60% or more of screened patients.

Doctors such as Barnett Kramer say that's cause for concern.

Kramer, the associate director for disease prevention at the National Institutes of Health, says CT scans—which take pictures of the whole chest—may pick up slow-growing cancers that do not pose a threat. Or they may find mysterious growths outside the lungs that may, or may not, alert doctors to real problems.

Benign lumps and bumps—which might never be detected without a CT scan—also may needlessly frighten patients, he says. Most questionable lesions are benign growths or scars from earlier infections, such as pneumonia or tuberculosis.

In light of this, the prevention task force announced there is not yet enough evidence to recommend for or against any kind of lung cancer screening.

Because CT screening for lung cancer is so new, doctors have not yet agreed how to handle suspicious test results. That creates a dilemma for doctors—and anxiety for patients, Lichtenfeld says.

Doctors may opt to wait to see whether the suspicious nodule grows. "Imagine if someone tells you, 'You have a nodule in your lung, but we want to wait three months before we do another scan,'" Lichtenfeld says.

Doctors also may test for cancer by taking a small tissue sample. But that can expose patients to invasive and potentially risky procedures, says Kramer, a member of the executive committee for the NCI trial.

Doctors retrieve lung tissue in different ways, depending on the location of the tumor. "None of these are pleasant," Kramer says.

Doctors may thread a thin, lighted tube into the mouth or nose to reach lesions in the center of the chest. To reach tumors on the lung's outer edges, they may insert a needle or scope through the chest, which risks collapsing the lung.

"The danger is that you're going through normal lung and airway to get to the tumor, and then you depend on the lung to seal itself off quickly," Kramer says.

In the worst cases, when suspected growths are located deep in the lungs, surgeons may opt to open the chest, Kramer says. The

procedure is painful and requires general anesthesia. Patients face
risks such as infection or fatal heart attacks.

Cautious About Procedures

Henschke says that doctors following careful guidelines perform
relatively few unnecessary biopsies. But Kramer notes that many
people who undergo these procedures will not have cancer. NCI
trial supervisors will carefully monitor mortality rates from all
causes, including complications that result from the screening tests.

Lichtenfeld says that doctors have learned to be cautious about
new procedures because of past mistakes.

In the 1990s, physicians gave bone-marrow transplants to breast
cancer patients, hoping that the women would improve, he says.
Controlled trials later showed that women got no benefit. Doctors
now rarely recommend the procedures for breast cancer.

"Just because you think something works better," Lichtenfeld
says, "doesn't mean it really works better."

Computed Tomography May Expose Children to Cancer Risk

By C.P. Kaiser

After years of improvements in standard X-ray technology, the levels of radiation needed to expose film have been cut dramatically, and with that reduction has come a lessening of health risk to patients. With the increasingly frequent use of computed tomography (CT) scans, however, the risk of genetic damage from X-ray exposure has re-emerged as an issue in medical imaging. In the selection below medical journalist C.P. Kaiser reviews the mounting evidence that CT scans may be putting children in danger. A single CT scan is safe, Kaiser says, but studies suggest that multiple scans during youth may lead to death from cancer later in life. One study predicts that of six hundred thousand children undergoing CT scans each year, five hundred will die of cancer as a direct result of their exposure to X-rays. A later study reduces the estimate to two hundred deaths, but even so, the study has led to public concern about CT safety, Kaiser claims. In response, medical practitioners, CT technology manufacturers, and the U.S. Food and Drug Administration have begun seeking ways to ensure safe doses. However, Kaiser writes, others in the field consider the dangers to have been exaggerated. C.P. Kaiser is a health journalist who regularly reports on medical imaging issues.

omen with scoliosis who as young girls routinely received multiple x-rays of the spine in the early to mid-20th century were found to have a significantly higher risk of breast cancer mortality as adults than the general population. Although current x-ray techniques use considerably lower doses of radiation the exposure from a routine multidetector CT [computed tomography] exam (5 to 20 rad) is just as high.[1]

The *Spine* study reported that the risk of breast cancer mortality increased with the number of x-rays and with cumulative dose to the breast. The girls who received cumulative doses greater than 20 rad had a three times greater chance of dying from breast cancer. Many children today receive multiple CT scans, easily topping a 20-rad ceiling.

For many years, radiation exposure during routine x-ray exams seemed a nonissue because radiation levels could be noted by looking at the film; a dark film, for example, meant too much radiation. Then CT was introduced.

Risk of Cancer

Unlike x-ray, CT scanning produces exceptional images at higher doses. Radiologists have assumed that the risk of cancer from CT radiation exposure is necessary, negligible, or both. The truth, say a growing number of experts, is that repeated pediatric spiral CT exams, especially those done at adult exposure levels, pose a cancer risk that can no longer be ignored. Children are particularly vulnerable because they are inherently more radiosensitive than adults and have more time to express cancers.

"It is clear that pediatric CT is different from adult CT, and also from any other radiological exam," said David J. Brenner, Ph.D., a radiobiologist at the Center for Radiological Research at Columbia University. "The organ doses are higher for children than for adults, and pediatric CT is increasing more rapidly than adult CT."

Almost everyone agrees that the benefit from any one CT scan outweighs the risk. But collectively, the risk from several million pediatric scans—often several in the same patient—represents a long-term public health problem, according to Eric J. Hall, Ph.D., director of the Center for Radiological Research. In their seminal paper published in the *American Journal of Roentgenology* [*AJR*], Brenner, Hall, and colleagues concluded that of the 600,000 children who undergo abdominal and head CT scans annually in the

---

1. A rad is a standard measure of ionizing (high-energy) radiation absorbed by the body.

U.S., 500 might ultimately die from cancer attributable to the CT radiation.

In a more recent paper, Brenner based his estimates on a dose of 200 mAs rather than 400 mAs, as the former is more representative of today's scanning parameters.[2] The new estimates also reduce by half the expected number of deaths attributable to CT radiation. Of those 600,000 children scanned each year, approximately 140,00 will ultimately die of cancer anyway. The projection of 200 CT-related deaths represents a small percentage increase over this background, he said.

"It's not an issue for an individual parent; rather, it's an issue for radiologists," Brenner said.

Public Concern

Despite the intentions of Brenner and his colleagues, *USA Today* and *Time* magazine picked up the story and made it a public issue. Since that time, several organizations, particularly the Society for Pediatric Radiology, have waged a campaign to educate pediatric and general radiologists, referring physicians, manufacturers, and government officials about pediatric CT dose management.

"A multidisciplinary approach is the best and only way to address this issue," said Dr. Thomas A. Slovis, radiology chief at Children's Hospital of Michigan and U.S. editor-elect of *Pediatric Radiology*.

To that end, Slovis has enlisted scientists, physicians, and vendors to brainstorm on short- and long-term solutions for optimizing pediatric imaging while minimizing dose. Medical physicists have suggested using uniform dose terminology; radiologists and technologists would like to see the exact dose, not an estimate, appear on the scanner; technologists want the dosage automatically adjusted for patient size and mass; and epidemiologists recommend that scanners archive dose information for tracking purposes. The FDA [U.S. Food and Drug Administration] is considering revising its CT standards, implemented before the advent of multidetector scanning, and manufacturers are researching ways to improve beam hardening, collimation, and detector absorption.

Implementing these ideas can be difficult, however. CT dose vernacular, for example, varies among engineers, radiologists, and

---

2. mAs are milliampere-seconds, a standard measure of the output of an X-ray machine.

manufacturers—and changes again across the Atlantic. Standardizing radiation dose calculation is another problem. Because the
body's organs and tissues vary in their susceptibility to cancer,
medical physicists have devised an average whole-body absorbed
rate called the effective dose. Even though "effective dose" and
"dose" are often used interchangeably, they are not the same.
Many physicists believe the effective dose is 10% to 25% lower
than the actual dose.

"People see a low effective dose readout and are satisfied, but it
is not the actual dose amount," Brenner said. "Either people need
to be aware of this, or we need a more accurate measurement."

Manufacturers, by FDA mandate, provide the CT dose index
(CTDI), which calculates the scanner's radiation output and absorption in phantoms.[3] As CT technology has advanced, physicists
have introduced several nonregulatory index variants, such as
CTDI100, CTDIw, and CTDIvol, which they say have broader applications and/or more utility.

"The bottom line is that these variants have replaced the FDA
definition of CTDI," said Stanley H. Stern, Ph.D., a health physicist at the FDA's Center for Devices and Radiological Health. "As
a result, there is confusion among CT users about precise defini-
tions of CTDI values."

Despite this confusion, there is general consensus on three facts:
- CT scanners produce much more radiation than conventional
  film x-ray;
- Children are more radiosensitive than adults, girls more so
  than boys, and they absorb a higher effective dose per organ;
  and
- The use of spiral CT is increasing even faster in children than
  in adults.

Children at Greater Risk

What everyone does not agree on is the danger, if any, this might
pose. In the past, statistics on the risk from small doses of radiation were extrapolations from high-dose exposures. That is no
longer the case as data from atomic bomb survivors have matured,
Hall said. These data indicate that young children are at least 10

---

3. Phantoms, in radiology jargon, are inorganic substitutes for human tissues used to estimate
radiation absorption.

times more sensitive than adults to radiation-induced malignancies. Atomic bomb survivors who received low-level radiation doses comparable to those associated with MD [multidetector] CT scans show a slightly higher incidence of cancer mortality.

"No theories, no assumptions, no extrapolations, and no models are involved. The risks are no longer speculative. They've been directly measured in a human population," Hall said last year [2002] at a symposium sponsored by the National Council on Radiation Protection and Measurement (NCRP) and the National Cancer Institute.

Some See Lower Risk

Not everyone agrees with Hall and Brenner's methods or conclusions. Critics argue that data from atomic bomb survivors are only estimates that do not accurately reflect real-time data from CT scanners, and a one-time whole-body exposure (as received by atomic bomb survivors) differs significantly from therapeutic partial-body doses. Dr. Michael N. Brant-Zawadzki, radiology chair at Hoag Memorial Hospital in Newport Beach, CA, cites the American College of Radiology's 1996 publication, *Radiation Risk: A Primer*, which states that an assumption of low-dose risk gleaned from high-dose exposure is a crude approximation. There is no evidence in favor of that assumption, or against it, according to the primer.

Another point on which Brant-Zawadzki and others disagree with Brenner et al is their use of the linear nonthreshold hypothesis, which claims that any level of radiation exposure, no matter how small, automatically increases one's cancer risk. In the November issue of *AJR*, Bernard L. Cohen, Ph.D., a professor emeritus of physics at the University of Pittsburgh, presents emerging information that questions the nonthreshold theory. He concludes that the theory fails in the low-dose region because it grossly overestimates the risk from low-level radiation. But Slovis called Cohen's data dated, citing the NCRP report, *Evaluation of the Linear Nonthreshold Dose Response Model for Nonionizing Radiation*, which found no evidence against the linear nonthreshold theory and concluded that it should stand.

Dr. Robert L. Brent, a professor of pediatrics, radiology, and pathology at Alfred I. duPont Hospital for Children in Wilmington, DE, said that the hypothesis is appropriate for establishing maximum permissible exposures for genotoxic [gene-damaging] environmental agents, including ionizing radiation, but may not be appropriate for accurately predicting the incidence of cancer in all CT-exposed children. Brent advocates an epidemiological study of children who have undergone multiple CT scans over time. Those data would more accurately reflect the risk than data from atomic bomb survivors who were exposed to one large dose of gamma rays, he said.

"To know the true risk of CT exposure, we need to study people who have had CT scans," Brent said. "We need to start now with an epidemiological program."

FDA Reviews the Standards

Since Brenner et al posited the danger of pediatric spiral CT scans, the FDA has been reexamining its standard for dose documentation. The CTDI standard was enacted 20 years ago and doesn't adequately address multidetector scanning.

Possible amendments to the current regulations would require standardizing dose indices and requiring scanners to display and record dose exposure. Standardized indices would be based on reference dose values, a concept introduced in the U.K. about 10 years ago and now making its way into the U.S.

In its new CT accreditation program, for example, the ACR requires facility audits of dose values for comparison with reference levels. According to one estimate by Stern at the CDRH, the systematic use of dose-index display or recording in a facility audit program could reduce patient CT dose by 15%.

Another new mandate under consideration would require scanners to be equipped with automatic exposure control systems, potentially reducing patient CT dose by 30%, according to Stern. Manufacturers have already introduced several automated approaches that span a range of technical complexity. At one end are systems offering recommendations for specified technique settings for tube current (mAs) and voltage (kVp) that the user may choose to apply. At the other end, the CT system continuously updates mAs and kVp in three dimensions based on measurements of x-ray attenuation. In between these two extremes are several other algorithms that offer, for example, automated tube current modulation axially for various image qualities a user may select.

Although these equipment features may be technically feasible,

the following questions remain, according to Stern:
- Would the dose index be based on average values for all models of scanners, or would it be specific to a particular unit?
- Should the displayed or recorded dose index be based on real-time measurements made during actual patient examinations?
- Regarding automatic exposure control, who defines the optimal amounts of radiation needed by the detectors for particular imaging tasks: manufacturers, radiologists, or the FDA?
- Would malpractice concerns increase with the possibility of associating recorded values with patient medical records?

Seeking Acceptable Parameters

Operators of today's CT scanners must look at the big picture in terms of dose reduction. Many parameters contribute to excessive dose, including mAs, kVp, pitch, slice thickness, detector efficiency, and patient size. Given that a modern scanner offers more than 400 possible combinations to reduce dose, what are harried radiologists to do?

"Practicing radiologists want the academic community to define a range of acceptable scanning parameters within which they will work," said Dr. Donald Frush, division chief of pediatric radiology at Duke University.

At Children's Hospital in Cincinnati, all CT scanning areas display pediatric weight-based charts that are broken down into seven sections each for the chest and abdomen. While the kVp [voltage] remains static at 120, the mAs is adjusted accordingly. Breast shields are routinely used for girls, whether the chest or the abdomen is scanned, said Dr. Lane Donnelly, associate director of radiology. Donnelly has forwarded these charts to colleagues.

Frush has instituted a nine-part color-coded dose-reduction chart for various pediatric sizes. He suggests that manufacturers equip scanners with a display that shows the results of dose adjustments. As radiologists tweak dose parameters for a lower setting, they could see in real-time what happens to image quality. He also wants radiologists to participate in and promote the ACR CT accreditation program.

"Our goal traditionally has been to get the best pictures possible. We no longer need to think that way." Frush said. "We have to start thinking in terms of thresholds for detection and allowing suboptimal image quality."

General radiologists, who perform about 85% of pediatric scans, are a focus of the current education campaign, as are referring physicians and other hospital personnel. Some educators have proposed that all personnel who meet with patients be able to describe the estimated radiation dose and relative risk of a CT scan. Others consider this unreasonable, and believe it might cause undue fear. The Mayo Clinic in Rochester, MN, gives all patients a brochure that describes the risk of every radiological procedure.

Training May Focus on CT Risks

The American Society of Radiological Technologists is considering developing individualized training modules for initial education in CT. Comprising both didactic and clinical components, the modules would focus on patient assessment, radiation physics, radiation protection, and examination protocols.

"The majority of CT techs in the U.S. were educated and certified as radiographers and then trained on the job to operate CT equipment. As CT evolves, so must the education of technologists," said Anne M. Edwards, who represented the ASRT at the NCRP/NCI symposium.

Although the danger of relatively low levels of CT radiation exposure is controversial, many feel it's prudent to err on the side of caution. In a commentary in *AJR*, Edward L. Nickoloff, D.Sc., chief hospital physicist at Columbia Presbyterian Medical Center, and Dr. Philip O. Alderson, radiology chair at the same institution, recommended special attraction to pediatric and thoracic CT when the field-of-view includes the female breasts.

They suggested that radiologists take leadership roles in the control of radiation exposure from diagnostic CT. Ultimately, dose management is the responsibility of the radiologist signing off on the study, according to Nickoloff and Alderson.

The Rising Cost of Medical Imaging Causes Concern

By Mike Norbut

Physicians who feel their incomes have been squeezed by reduced reimbursements from health insurers and the government are increasingly turning to medical imaging as a supplementary source of income. In the following selection medical reporter Mike Norbut explains that some large physicians' groups have invested in their own high-tech imaging equipment, such as MRI machines, to make extra income from their patients. This has contributed to a rapid rise in health-care costs related to medical imaging. Health insurers and government agencies have responded with a variety of moves aimed at curbing the growth of medical imaging procedures. Some insurers have begun to require an opportunity to approve or veto a doctor's referral for medical imaging. More than half of the states have passed laws requiring certificates of need to justify reimbursements from government health programs for medical imaging equipment. Some physicians object to the paperwork and delays these constraints impose, Norbut reports. Others worry that the need to cut costs will prompt doctors to purchase inferior equipment, thereby reducing the quality of imaging that patients receive. There is consensus, however, that needless medical imaging should be stopped. Mike Norbut is a Chicago-based staff writer for the *American Medical News*. He frequently covers issues related to health-care costs.

Ancillary revenue has become a key to financial survival for many physicians in a world of declining reimbursements. For some larger groups, the strategy has revolved around

Mike Norbut, "MRI Backlash: Crackdown on Costs of Imaging," *American Medical News,* vol. 47, December 6, 2004, p. 15. Copyright © 2004 by the American Medical Association. Reproduced by permission.

MRI machines and other imaging equipment—high-ticket items that carry the potential for profitability.

While it has a hefty price tag, in-office imaging equipment has proven to be a convenient option for patients and a positive investment for physicians, so it's no wonder that many groups would want to add that service to their repertoire.

The revenue stream, however, is not without its share of dams, as insurers and government agencies look to rein in costs. Overutilization, especially when it comes to imaging, has become a hot-button topic in health care, and physicians are finding the decision to purchase an MRI machine to be about more than whether they can afford it.

They also have to consider if they'll get paid for the tests.

"In the whole debate of imaging equipment in offices, whether you agree or disagree, ultimately [insurers] have the trump card," said James Borgstede, MD, a radiologist in Colorado Springs, Colo., and chair of the board of chancellors of the American College of Radiology. "If they see it as a problem, they're going to solve the problem."

The problem, as defined by insurers and the Medicare Payment Advisory Commission, is the rapid growth of diagnostic imaging tests. In a March [2004] report to Congress, MedPAC said imaging utilization grew faster than any other physician service, at 9.4%, between 2001 and 2002. Some types of imaging, such as nuclear medicine and advanced MRI, grew more than 17%, according to the report.

Likewise, Pittsburgh-based Highmark BlueCross BlueShield said its spending on imaging claims had increased 20% annually over the last three years.

Pressure on Physicians

In response, Highmark is launching a new program focused on reprivileging [renewal of eligibility for payment] physicians in its network who perform imaging services and requiring preauthorization for imaging procedures. The insurer hopes the idea of limiting contracts and implementing a more stringent referral policy will increase quality and bring imaging usage rates closer to the national average, said Carey Vinson, MD, Highmark's medical director for quality management.

Similarly, Harvard Pilgrim Health Care, based in Wellesley,

Mass., started a preauthorization program in July. Practices are required to submit information to National Imaging Associates, a radiology utilization management firm based in New Jersey, before ordering a test. About 10% of the time, doctors end up having to discuss the case with a National Imaging Associates representative, who may suggest a different course of action instead of the imaging test, Harvard Pilgrim officials said.

The tactics affect more than just radiologists. Cardiology, orthopedics and neurology are some of the other specialties that have embraced imaging technology in their own offices. While the practice is not yet widespread among insurers, the idea of health plans taking it upon themselves to try to get a handle on costs is not surprising to many physicians.

"I think it's absolutely justified," said James Donaldson, MD, radiologist-in-chief of the Dept. of Medical Imaging at Children's Memorial Hospital in Chicago. "Clearly, the federal government won't be able to modify Stark laws soon enough to suit insurers."[1]

States Impose Restrictions

Certainly, the insurers' clampdown can create a situation in which professional rivalries are bound to come out, especially between radiologists and nonradiologists.

Rather than battle with insurers, physician groups in some states end up battling each other for the chance to gain access to the MRI revenue stream.

Some 36 states have certificate-of-need laws, which were in place before health plans started looking at their own cost-limiting measures. They usually target expensive health care items, such as imaging machines or new construction, and they're theoretically meant to keep utilization rates from running out of control.

In North Carolina, for example, eight separate entities—including five physician groups—are vying for the approval to purchase one MRI machine for Wake County. The state takes an inventory of machines and the number of procedures performed by them in each region and weighs that number against its own capacity determinations to decide if a need for more machines exists, said Mike McKillip, project analyst for the Certificate of Need Section

---

1. "Stark laws" are federal laws restricting physicians from making patient referrals where conflicts of interest may arise.

of the North Carolina Dept. of Health and Human Services.

Not only is it a nerve-racking ordeal to wait for a decision, but the application process is an expensive one, said W. Kent Davis, MD, a radiologist and president of Raleigh Radiology, which has a hospital location and three stand-alone offices.

"I understand the rationale for why they have [a CON law (certificate of need)]," Dr. Davis said. "Would it be nice to go out and buy an MRI without asking permission? Yes. But doctors need to realize we need to be responsible for how we contribute to health care costs."

Incentives for Overuse

Part of Dr. Donaldson's role with Children's Memorial Hospital is to oversee the selection and purchase of MRIs and other imaging machines. Over the years, the hospital has made some expensive capital investments in hopes of raising the bar for pediatric care.

It's easy to make a recommendation for high-quality equipment when the hospital is spending the money, Dr. Donaldson said. But in today's economic environment, doctors in private practice might not be so willing to make such a deep financial commitment. Or, they even might buy a cheaper machine and perform lower-quality scans as a result he said.

"I think it is risky," said Dr. Donaldson, a radiologist who said his group, a 16-physician subsidiary of the hospital, has talked conceptually with Children's about investing in imaging machines as a joint venture. "If I'm just an entrepreneur looking to invest some money, I would be a little leery."

Entrepreneurial spirit is one of the reasons behind overutilization, Dr. Borgstede said. Ordering tests with revenue in the back of your mind can add unnecessary cost to the system, he said.

Radiologists, insurers and government agencies alike have said nonradiologists bear some of the responsibility for increasing utilization rates because of the equipment they purchase for their own offices. A worst-case reimbursement scenario, Dr. Borgstede said, is that insurers decide to cut costs by simply cutting their conversion factor.

"If you're in the business to make money, you increase your utilization again, and then you're paid half as much again," Dr. Borgstede said. "Pretty soon, they will achieve cost savings, but the way they do it is horrible for my business. The only thing I do in medicine is imaging. After the shambles are created, I'm the one who's left to pick it up."

Nonradiologists say there are definite benefits to having in-office imaging equipment, with better quality and patient convenience topping the list. The American Academy of Orthopaedic Surgeons, for example, takes the position that orthopedists are qualified to perform imaging studies and interpret results, and the limitation strategy by insurers "undermines both the quality and convenience" of patient care.

"Patients want a timely diagnosis," said Robert H. Haralson III, MD, executive director of medical affairs for AAOS. Dr. Haralson recently left a 42-physician group in Knoxville, Tenn., that owns three MRI machines to join the academy. "If you have a patient in your office, you want to be able to x-ray them right there. If I take a cast off and say, 'OK, you have to go across town,' they're going to raise so much Cain that the insurance company will have to give in," he said.

For cardiologists, the issue centers on nuclear imaging, which is a growing in-office service. The test is a vital tool for diagnosing the level of heart disease in a patient, and cardiologists are the best-trained physicians in interpreting the results, said Michael Wolk, MD, president of the American College of Cardiology and professor of clinical medicine at Weill Medical College at Cornell University in New York.

"If evidence-based medicine is being used, I think you will see an increase in utilization, and it will save many dollars by helping cardiologists to make better diagnoses early," Dr. Wolk said.

Quality Counts

Diagnostic testing saves money, physicians maintain, when the tests are performed by high-quality machines. Relatively speaking, there are some inexpensive MRI machines available that render inconclusive results, requiring follow-up scans and more cost, doctors said.

"If they made a rule, which makes sense to me, that no scan of a brain or spine should be done on a machine with less than a 1.5 tesla magnet, that would change things immediately," said James J. Anthony, MD, a neurologist with Riverhills Healthcare Inc, a multispecialty practice in Cincinnati. Dr. Anthony and his partners own a 1.5 tesla MRI machine, which produces a magnetic field

30,000 times stronger than the earth's own magnetic field. The stronger the magnet, the higher quality the image. "I tried talking to insurance companies about this 10 or 15 years ago, but they didn't care," he said.

Physicians agree that a key to the imaging debate is using quality to weed out the facilities that could be contributing to increasing costs by ordering tests based on their bottom line.

Dr. Wolk, for example, said he supports the credentialing of nuclear laboratories, and the ACC is working to educate cardiologists about imaging utilization guidelines and the ethics of appropriate self-referral. Dr. Borgstede said the American College of Radiology was not pushing a Stark-style legislation package, but this also isn't the time for physicians to wait and see how payers react to growing costs.

Setting quality benchmarks would ensure that the proper physicians are performing and reading the scans. It would protect patients better, and it would keep costs down, he said.

"I don't think the status quo is going to continue," Dr. Borgstede said. "In some fashion, all insurers will deal with this, and clearly, they have articulated to us that it's a problem. Optimally, for us, we'll be able to engage other specialties in a dialogue and find out what is the appropriate way to deal with utilization."

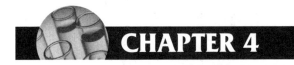

CHAPTER 4

Emerging Applications in Medical Imaging

Computed Tomography for the Heart

By Cinda Becker

The application of computed tomography to diagnose heart disease has resulted in a new imaging specialty: cardiovascular computed tomography (CT). In the following selection health-care journalist Cinda Becker describes how CT differs from conventional heart imaging, and how its introduction has touched off conflict between cardiologists and radiologists. A key difference between the two diagnostic techniques is that conventional diagnostic catheterization, better known as angiography, requires the insertion of a long tube into the heart whereas the CT scan is noninvasive. Cardiologists are anxious to avoid reductions in angiography procedures, which only they are qualified to perform, while radiologists, whose expertise is in imaging technologies, are eager to expand the use of CT scans for the heart. Becker reports that a battle between the two kinds of specialists over use of these technologies is brewing. Additionally, questions about the costs, both for patients and for society, have arisen. As more patients elect to undergo expensive CT scans, medical costs will rise. Cinda Becker is New York bureau chief for *Modern Healthcare.* In May 2003 she won the National Institute for Health Care Management's annual award for excellence in health-care reporting.

Haunted by a family history of heart disease and uneasily facing his 50th birthday, Alan Muney couldn't resist the offer to undergo a cardiac computed tomography [CT] test that his employer, Oxford Health Plans, in most cases won't pay for.

Muney, executive vice president and chief medical officer of the insurer, never experienced any symptoms of heart disease, but his father suffered a massive heart attack when he was 45 years old and died at 49. Both his grandfathers also died of heart disease. Muney has been under a cardiologist's care and was considering another stress test, which he had passed with flying colors in the past, but a radiologist colleague suggested a CT angiography instead. Though not well accepted by cardiologists yet, "the radiology community believes it is going to be the up-and-coming thing, so I volunteered," Muney says.

Some cardiologists may view this new technology as a Trojan horse, commandeered by radiologists prepared to steal away their business—if they don't steal it from the radiologists first. CT is growing increasingly adept at quickly capturing three-dimensional X-ray images, and there is little doubt that it will eventually become a key diagnostic tool in detecting life-threatening plaque buildup in the coronary arteries. The only question is when. Certainly it is not expected until public programs and private payers uniformly reimburse for it.

"I don't think it's quite ready for prime time," says Barry Katzen, an interventional radiologist who is founder and medical director of the Miami (Fla.) Cardiac and Vascular Institute at 551-bed Baptist Hospital of Miami. "We're very excited about it. It is definitely going to change the paradigm of how the coronary arteries are looked at."

A Noninvasive Alternative

When it does become a standard, it is still uncertain whether CT angiography as a screening tool will become yet another cost layer or a substitution for existing technologies. Some such as Muney predict it will replace, upstream, the standard stress test, a nuclear-based physiological test that is ubiquitous in cardiologists' offices but tends to produce a lot of false-positive results. Others such as Katzen say they believe that, downstream, it will eventually offer a patient-friendly substitution for diagnostic cardiac catheterization,[1] also known as coronary angiography, a lucrative invasive procedure for peeking into coronary arteries that helps fortify the bottom line of hospitals that offer it. (Magnetic resonance imag-

1. an X-ray procedure in which a thin tube inserted through an artery releases dye in the heart as the image is taken

ing also is quickly becoming a standard for noninvasive imaging of the peripheral areas of the cardiovascular system, but cardiologists are less likely to co-opt it because of the technology's sophistication and cost.)

Discarding diagnostic catheterization in favor of CT angiography could be an economic boon for hospitals as long as they are prepared to mediate the inevitable battles between cardiologists and radiologists. The noninvasive, diagnostic alternative to cardiac catheterization can screen patients in a fraction of the time and could free staff-intensive catheterization laboratory space. . . .

Specialists at Odds

Although no one who has survived the reportedly bruising disagreements is eager to talk about it, stories about turf wars between radiologists and cardiologists have been legion. Indeed, radiologists were once the proprietors of stress testing and cardiac catheterization until cardiologists co-opted those modalities, says Stephen Koch, medical director of Imaging Heart, a New York–based company that offers cardiac CT, relying heavily on referrals from cardiology groups. Cardiologists can easily justify the need to oversee a stress test in case something goes awry for the patient, and it's a relatively inexpensive technology to install in a private practice. For many of the same reasons, radiologists would want a cardiologist on hand when performing a cardiac catheterization, Koch says.

"There are going to be huge turf wars," Koch says. "What's different now is that CT imaging is the bread and butter of radiology groups."

Cardiologists first put nuclear stress testing in their offices—for as much as $600,000—when hospitals barred them from reading the nuclear portions of the exams, says Karen Hartman, vice president of Corazon Consulting, a firm specializing in cardiovascular programs. She estimates that as many as 80% of all cardiology offices have purchased the technology. Some cardiologists likewise will move to bring CT into their practices, but the winners in the end will be the hospitals that successfully bring the two specialties together, she says. Hospitals that allow the animosity to fester could face the same situation as a community hospital she left unnamed. A key radiology group left the facility after cardiologists exclusively were given peripheral vascular services, Hartman says.

There is not much time to deal with the issues: In the next few months [after December 2003] the 32-slice CT will be introduced, offering more detectors for even better resolution and speed, she notes.

Rapidly advancing multislice CT technology has paved the way for its inroads into the cardiovascular suite, especially the introduction of the 16-slice machine in 2002, says Bernd Ohnesorge, vice president of the CT division of Siemens Medical Solutions. The 16-slice CT, priced at approximately $1.2 million, offered image resolution and speed that made it conducive to capturing the small anatomy of a beating heart, from the arteries carrying life-giving blood to small lesions that could impede that flow. . . .

Business Factors Driving CT

The business case for cardiac CT is building, even if reimbursement is spotty at best. Image to image, CT has many advantages over diagnostic cardiac catheterization in patient turnaround. One CT machine can easily push through one patient every 15 minutes, Prather says. Meanwhile, catheterization labs at best can turn around about one patient per hour, he says.

However, if the coronary angiogram uncovers a problem requiring an intervention in the same setting—and as many as 70% of them do—"your schedule is blown for the day," Hickman says. "An interventional procedure can absorb 30% to 50% of the capacity of your cath lab," costing the hospital much-needed revenue if the catheterization laboratory's fixed resources aren't managed properly, he says.

Ultimately, taking the diagnostic procedures out of the catheterization lab to make more time for therapeutic procedures will bring in more revenue for the hospital, says DeAnn Haas, global marketing manager of cardiac CT for GE Medical Systems. Haas says most of GE's customers are radiologists purchasing cardiac applications for their multislice scanners. She estimates that 75% of the multislice scanners that are sold are leaving GE with cardiac applications built into them.

Still, the two-dimensional images provided by a diagnostic cardiac catheterization remain the gold standard, especially since CT could not replace subsequent interventional procedures, such as stenting, that might be needed as a result of the exam, Ohnesorge says. But in the next three to five years, he predicts technologies

will merge so that CT imaging also will become a part of interventional procedures. But correctly CT can "be an alternative in
a select group of patients for ruling out the presence of disease,"
he says.

Hickman says CT angiography would open the market to "a
whole new population"—between ages 35 and 45 with no symptoms but a family history of heart disease—who wouldn't consider
undergoing a diagnostic catheterization, knowing the high odds
of a problem being found.

Burden on Healthcare Costs

The potential new market raises questions regarding the new technology's cost, especially in light of a study released last month
[November 2003] that found that the more a technology is available, the more it gets used, fueling greater healthcare spending.
Of four areas examined in the study—cancer, cardiac and new-
born care and diagnostic imaging—the researchers found free-
standing diagnostic imaging had the strongest link between higher
availability and higher spending.

"There's always a potential that with new things like (CT angiography) the technology will get added on," says Laurence
Baker, the lead author of the study, which was released by the
journal *Health Affairs* and bankrolled by the Blue Cross and Blue
Shield Association. "Giving everyone a CT instead of a catheterization would look like a cost savings, but there is a dynamic aspect." The new market of patients Hickman describes could generate a lot of additional procedures, Baker notes. Then again, if
those additional procedures save lives "it all comes down to cost-
benefit," Baker says.

Comparison Study Under Way

A study examining the clinical and economic efficacy of screening cardiac patients with CT and other imaging modalities is under way at 905-bed Mount Sinai Medical Center in New York. Patients with no symptoms but a 20% or greater risk of suffering a
heart attack in the next 10 years are undergoing four different exams, including CT angiography and MRI. Valentin Fuster, director of Mount Sinai's cardiovascular institute, says as much as 10%
of the population over the age of 30 is in this risk group. The study

is funded by the National Institutes of Health and a consortium that includes imaging vendors.

Fuster says he is certain the technology will prove less expensive. CT angiography costs about $600 per procedure and about the same for MRI images, but costs can run to as much as $3,000 for a diagnostic catheterization, he says. "We cannot go into 10% of the population who don't have symptoms at all and do catheterization," Fuster says. "These noninvasive technologies are going to be incredibly important in the future."

Although trained as a cardiologist, Fuster brought MRI as a cardiac diagnostic technique to Mount Sinai, putting it in the radiology department because "radiologists have better infrastructure technologies," he says. But it's a technology "that needs to be shared" by both specialties, he says.

Mount Sinai never became the victim of turf battles because "we both realized that was a losing strategy," says Burton Drayer, Mount Sinai's chairman, professor of radiology and executive vice president of hospital and clinical affairs. "When you think in terms of turf, you think in terms of failure. No one wins a turf battle. . . . The winning strategy is for everybody to collaborate.". . .

More Screenings in the Future

As to whether earlier detection represents a win for the healthcare system as a whole, "that will be argued over the next 100 years," Drayer says. "I think society is requesting of us that we are able to look at them in a noninvasive manner and tell them whether anything is wrong, so I only see the numbers increasing as they become more health-conscious." It's a double-edged sword, he adds, because with more patients being screened, more patients are found to have something wrong, "and then you are forced to move on to the next step. . . . When you have almost miraculous techniques, you begin to see almost too much." Drayer says he "would hope" that by 2010, the typical cardiac catheterization will be therapeutic rather than diagnostic.

Katzen of the Miami Cardiac and Vascular Institute already is thinking about the day when CT technology fully arrives in cardiovascular suites, and when that happens, there will be "a tremendous impact," he says. For one, patients won't need cardiologists any longer for referrals; primary-care physicians and internists will be able to order the procedure. That scenario would seem to alienate cardiologists, but from the day the institute was opened in 1987, "we tried to build an infrastructure dedicated to the delivery of integrated cardiology care," he says. "The idea was to bring all the disciplines of care together—cardiologists, vascular surgeons, neurologists, nephrologists—all of whom participate. . . . We wanted to treat the cardiovascular system as a single system.". . .

Based on past experience with vascular imaging in noncoronary areas, Katzen says they know that less-invasive techniques such as CT angiography can replace about 70% of corresponding invasive procedures such as coronary angiography. "What we're looking at in terms of the future is to create teams of physicians that would involve cardiology and radiology," he says. Right now cardiologists are reading coronary angiograms, but "if images are acquired in another modality, my feeling is those people would be involved along with radiology in the interpretation. The question is going to be how to partner and I think here's where having a multidisciplinary environment helps," Katzen says. . . .

A Clean Bill of Health

Muney of Oxford says the images produced by his CT angiography "were unbelievable in terms of quality." The results gave him a clean bill of health and peace of mind. Still, he says he believes it should remain an elective procedure for the time being until guidelines are established to ensure that the technology does not become overused in the same way nuclear cardiology arguably has become now that most cardiologists have the wherewithal to provide it in their offices. When they have it, they use it more, Muney says, echoing the findings of Baker's study.

"It's a good example of how medicine continually pushes the envelope," Muney says.

Diagnosing Alzheimer's with PET

By Daniel Silverman and Gary Small

In positron emission tomography, or PET, a radioactive isotope is injected into a patient along with targeting molecules that direct it to the site of interest. The isotope emits positrons, which are annihilated on contact with nearby electrons (their precise opposites), resulting in flashes that can be detected and used to form images. In the following selection two doctors, Daniel Silverman and Gary Small, describe how PET was able to accurately diagnose a woman with memory problems where previous magnetic resonance scans had been unable to identify the source of her difficulties. The 53-year-old woman, identified as "Ms. A," had spent years in various clinics trying to discover what was wrong with her. She then entered the care of the University of California, Los Angeles (UCLA) Memory Clinic, where a PET scan helped determine that she was suffering from dementia, with a probable diagnosis of Alzheimer's disease.

This was not the first time PET proved useful in identifying dementia. Silverman and Small write that clinicians and researchers have been gaining considerable experience using PET in such diagnoses since the 1980s. The procedure adds to the cost of diagnosis, but the relief to patients and their families of not having to go through numerous inconclusive tests may offset this. Although PET does involve radiation, Silverman and Small say the risks from exposure are minimal. Daniel H.S. Silverman, who holds both medical and doctoral degrees, is head of the neuronuclear imaging unit at UCLA's medical center and is a faculty member in the university's pharmacology department. Gary W. Small is a physician who serves as UCLA's Parlow-Solomon Professor on Aging and as director of the university's Center on Aging.

Clinical identification and differential diagnosis of dementia is especially challenging in its early stages, partly because of the difficulty in distinguishing it from the mild decline in memory that can occur with normal aging and from mild cognitive manifestations of other neuropsychiatric conditions, such as depression. As reported by the U.S. Agency for Health Care Policy and Research in 1996, "Early recognition of the condition has important benefits," which is even more the case today, now that several medications for the treatment of Alzheimer's disease are available by prescription; however, "early-stage dementia is often unrecognized or misdiagnosed." This is especially unfortunate for dementias like Alzheimer's due to neurodegenerative disease, since patients potentially have the most to gain from effective therapies that intervene as early as possible in the course of progressive irreversible damage to brain tissue.

The University of California, Los Angeles, Memory Clinic is primarily directed toward serving patients with mild memory changes who frequently have not experienced sufficient cognitive losses to meet diagnostic criteria for dementia. The mission of the clinic is driven by clinicopathological studies of recent years indicating that a substantial portion of such individuals are actually suffering from the earliest manifestations of Alzheimer's disease and related dementias, while conventional methods for evaluating those patients are inadequate for making reliable diagnostic and prognostic assessments. During the same period, advances in dementia research have identified genetic and environmental factors that significantly increase the risk of developing neurodegenerative disease; moreover, it has become increasingly evident that measurement of regional cerebral metabolism through positron emission tomography (PET) sensitively detects such disease at the time of its earliest symptomatic expression, or even preclinically. Although new PET technologies are being developed to measure the concentration of amyloid plaques and neurofibrillary tangles, the pathognomonic [disease-causing] lesions of Alzheimer's disease, this technology is as yet [un]available in clinical settings. By contrast, PET measurements of cerebral glucose metabolism are clinically available; considerable evidence indicates their usefulness in the early diagnosis of dementia. The clinical case described illustrates the typical outcomes of a conventional evaluation process and the dementia evaluation process as it is carried out in our memory clinic.

A Difficult Case to Diagnose

Ms. A was a 53-year-old woman who came to the memory clinic with the chief complaint that it was "hard to put thoughts together." She reported a progressive decline in her memory abilities over the previous 4 years, for which she had undergone general medical, neurological, psychiatric, and formal neuropsychological evaluations. She had been variously diagnosed as having depression, migraines, fibromyalgia, attention deficit disorder, and posttraumatic stress disorder stemming from childhood abuse. Her medications included the selective serotonin reuptake inhibitor citalopram [an antidepressant] (40 mg/day for the previous 18 months), levothyroxine for hypothyroidism secondary to Hashimoto's thyroiditis [a thyroid condition], and estrogen-replacement therapy.

A review of Ms. A's records from an outside health organization revealed that her internist first noted a cognitive problem 2½ years earlier when he recorded "memory loss" of 1½ years' duration. At that time he also diagnosed depression, obtained laboratory screening test results, referred Ms. A to a neurologist, and scheduled her for a return visit in 6 weeks.

The next month, Ms. A, accompanied by her husband, had her first visit with the neurologist. He noted that a computerized tomographic scan of the brain and tests of her CSF [cerebrospinal fluid], obtained in the remote past for workup of headache, were unremarkable. Her examination was normal, except for her mental status: "She appeared anxious and hyperventilated at times." Her neurologist concluded, "Most of the patient's symptoms are likely psychiatrically based. She is currently in therapy and being treated. Nevertheless, because of the indication of deteriorated function at work, documented by her husband [with whom she ran a small restaurant], I would like to get [magnetic resonance imaging] MRI of the brain to rule out any frontal lobe disease."

An MRI of her brain performed without contrast the next week showed a normal cortex, brainstem, basal ganglia, thalami, and ventricles. . . .

Two and one-half months after the second MRI, Ms. A returned to her internist, who noted, "Memory lapses persist." His plan was to follow up with the neurologist, refer Ms. A to the behavioral health unit, and have her return in 6 weeks. When she returned 6 weeks later, the internist again noted that "Memory lapses persist," and his assessment was "depression" and "memory loss.". . .

After another 6 months (1 year after Ms. A's first visit to the internist for memory loss), she returned to her internist, who again noted, "Memory lapses persist." His assessment indicated, "1) Hypothyroidism, 2) depression, 3) fibromyalgia."

Eight and one-half months later, Ms. A's husband brought her to a licensed psychologist for formal neuropsychological testing, again expressing the concern that his wife was "experiencing cognitive problems." Ms. A told the psychologist that she was afraid she was losing her mental capacity: "I forget things, I forget people I meet, lose things in my mind." The psychologist reported that Ms. A's verbal IQ was in the normal range, but her performance IQ was markedly deficient. The psychologist's summary stated, "The results suggest neurological difficulties, it can be said that posttraumatic stress disorder factors into the results. . . . However, neurological problems should be ruled out ASAP," and he further recommended individual counseling, as well as marriage counseling, because of "her concern for her husband's feelings about her difficulties."

Evaluation at the Memory Clinic

After another 9½ months, still without a specific diagnosis for her memory complaints, Ms. A was evaluated for the first time by a geriatric psychiatrist at the memory clinic. At her psychiatric examination, Ms. A was reported to be "alert, mildly anxious, euthymic, friendly, cooperative, with bright affect." Her performance on the Mini Mental State Examination (MMSE), however, was clearly abnormal; she scored only 18 of a possible 30 points and remembered none of three possible items for short-term recall. Once her previous brain imaging studies had been reviewed, a PET scan, which images regional brain metabolism with the use of fluorodeoxyglucose (FDG) [a radioactive agent], was obtained. The scan revealed diffuse and moderately severe cortical hypometabolism, especially affecting the bilateral midparietal cortex and left inferior frontal and temporal cortex, but sparing the bilateral sensorimotor and visual cortices. The nuclear medicine physician who interpreted the results noted that this pattern is characteristic of neurodegenerative dementia—most commonly, Alzheimer's disease. . . .

A week after the PET, a neuropsychologist administered a test battery to Ms. A and concluded that although "other diagnoses that she has received in the past, such as fibromyalgia, attention deficit disorder, posttraumatic stress disorder, and depression could be a factor in her performance, it is emphasized that they would not explain the severity or scope of her current deficits."

Successful Diagnosis and Treatment

The psychiatrist who originally saw Ms. A diagnosed probable Alzheimer's disease, citing the results of PET and neuropsychologic testing, as well as her unremarkable MRI. Treatment was initiated. . . . The family was also referred to the Alzheimer's Association for education and support and was informed that Ms. A should refrain from driving. She responded well to the treatment: her MMSE score increased from 18 to 21, and she correctly remembered two of three items on the test of short-term recall. Her husband described her as "more engaging with others, more alert." Ms. A and her husband decided to move to northern California to be closer to their children and to return to Los Angeles every 6 to 12 months for visits to the memory clinic.

To summarize Ms. A's clinical course, 4 years after she had onset of cognitive symptoms, and after 2½ years of conventional clinical workup for dementia (including multiple visits with her primary care physician, ongoing care with her psychiatrist, two visits to a neurologist, two MRI scans, and formal neuropsychological testing), she still had no specific diagnosis to explain her memory problems and was accordingly receiving no specific therapy for her dementia symptoms. Furthermore, she and her husband were offered no sense of the prognosis for her disorder or meaningful support for her condition.

By contrast, just 1 month after she came to the memory clinic, a diagnostic PET scan had been acquired, which demonstrated findings characteristic of neurodegenerative dementia, probably Alzheimer's disease. Neuropsychological testing a week later corroborated this diagnosis, and subsequent MRI ruled out other causes. On this new clinical path, appropriate pharmacotherapy was initiated, and Ms. A showed signs of improvement. In addition, she was linked up with useful community resources and began to formulate, with her husband, meaningful plans for themselves and their family.

Ms. A's young age may have contributed to some of the diagnostic delay. Most cases of Alzheimer's disease occur after age 65 years, while frontotemporal dementia more often has an onset in people in their 50s and 60s. A PET scan is useful in differentiating these two dementias . . .

Limits of MRI

Conventional MRI or computerized tomography of patients with symptoms of dementia may be useful in identifying unsuspected clinically significant lesions, which are present in approximately 5% of patients. However, they are nondiagnostic in patients with Alzheimer's-related pathophysiologic changes, which are much more common. Such scans are typically read as normal or as demonstrating only the nonspecific finding of cortical atrophy or, worst still, as revealing ischemic changes that are often misinterpreted as pointing to cerebrovascular disease as the primary or sole process responsible for the patient's cognitive decline. This, in turn, leads to failure to institute appropriate pharmacotherapy (i.e., tacrine, donepezil, rivastigmine, and galantamine—all of which are approved by the Food and Drug Administration only for the indication of "mild to moderate dementia of the Alzheimer's type"). It is unfortunately not rare for that type of misinterpretation to occur, even among expert clinicians. In a multicenter study involving seven university-affiliated Alzheimer's Disease Diagnostic and Treatment Centers, of the patients who were diagnosed after clinical and structural neuroimaging evaluations as having "vascular dementia" and in whom Alzheimer's disease and other dementia diagnoses were specifically thought to be absent, only 30% actually had isolated cerebrovascular disease, and the majority (55%) had Alzheimer's disease, as ascertained by pathological diagnosis.

Over the last two decades, clinicians and researchers have obtained substantial experience in using PET for the identification and differential diagnosis of dementia. Thousands of patients with clinically diagnosed and, in some cases, histopathologically [by examination of tissue under microscope] confirmed Alzheimer's disease from many independent laboratories have been studied by using PET measures of cerebral blood flow and glucose and oxygen use. . . . Blind clinical evaluations of PET scans can differentiate patients with Alzheimer's disease from patients with other dementias and from cognitively intact persons.

Studies comparing neuropathological examination with PET imaging, as with clinical assessment, are most informative in assessing diagnostic value. In the largest such single-institution series, [John M.] Hoffman and co-workers studied 22 patients with various types of dementia (including 64% with Alzheimer's disease alone and 9% with Alzheimer's disease plus additional neurological disease, who were identified by pathological diagnosis). Visual interpretation of scans, made by readers who were blinded to clinical information, yielded estimates of sensitivity and specificity for identifying the presence of Alzheimer's disease (88%–93% and 63%–67%, respectively). More recently, a multicenter study compared dementia diagnosis by using FDG PET with neuropathological diagnosis. The investigators collected data from an international consortium of clinical facilities, which had acquired both brain FDG PET and histopathological data for patients undergoing evaluation for dementia. Images and pathological data were independently classified as positive or negative for presence of a progressive neurodegenerative disease in general and Alzheimer's disease specifically. The PET results identified patients with Alzheimer's disease and patients with any neurodegenerative disease with a sensitivity of 94% in both cases . . . , and overall accuracies of 88% and 92%.

As suggested by pertinent literature, diagnostic workups that do not include such assessments of cerebral metabolism tend to be substantially less sensitive in the diagnosis of Alzheimer's disease. . . .

Costs and Benefits

With a preponderance of evidence clearly pointing to greater accuracy when FDG PET is incorporated into the diagnostic algorithm for evaluation of early dementia, the focus turns to the issue of whether it is worth the cost of getting this added information. Apart from financial considerations, several ramifications of having available the added information provided by PET bear upon this issue. For example, if accurate positive diagnoses were achieved early on, patients and their families could be spared the repeated batteries of diagnostic tests performed over extended periods of time, and they and their physicians would less often experience the frustrations of ambiguous diagnostic conclusions. The information would also enhance the ability of families to plan for issues pertinent to future patient care. This is particularly so in light of recent data indicating that the degree of hypometabolism identified by PET in certain affected brain regions predicts the rate of decline in standardized measures of memory that takes place in the years subsequent to PET examination.

Although PET offers a clear benefit in diagnostic accuracy above the standard clinical examination, errors in specificity still occur, raising concern for overdiagnosis of Alzheimer's disease. In our previous studies, many patients inaccurately diagnosed as having Alzheimer's disease instead had dementia with Lewy bodies or vascular or mixed dementia. Recent evidence indicates that cholinesterase inhibitor drugs, the currently approved treatment for Alzheimer's disease, also benefit these other dementias, minimizing the concern for such overdiagnosis. An additional risk is the psychological impact of the family learning of an Alzheimer's disease diagnosis. The greater sensitivity and benefits of early recognition and treatment offset such risks, and the better specificity with PET than with clinical evaluation alone actually decreases the chance of a false positive diagnosis.

In a critical review of the clinical value of neuroimaging in the diagnosis of dementia, it was pointed out that the total charges associated with performance of a dedicated brain PET amount to less than the cost of 1 year of unnecessary pharmacotherapy for treatment of a misdiagnosed patient or to 1 month of lost productivity. We recently completed a test of the extent to which the additional costs of scanning would be offset by the savings of improved diagnostic accuracy, employing the formalized tools of decision analysis. On the basis of accuracy estimates of clinical evaluation and PET reported in the literature and conservative estimates of savings realized, it was found that the added diagnostic accuracy obtained by incorporation of FDG PET into the routine clinical evaluation of patients seen with early symptoms of dementia could be achieved in an economically practical manner. In fact, the attendant improvement in accuracy allowed PET scans to essentially pay for themselves. A range-of-cost analysis indicated that the overall expense of management of patients seen with early dementia would be somewhat lower when PET was routinely incorporated, for all reimbursed costs of brain PET lower than approximately $2,700. (The amount that is currently reimbursed for brain PET is typically over $1,000 less than that figure.)

Risks Are Low

The PET scanning procedure is well tolerated by the vast majority of patients; the risks involve minimal radiation exposure. For identifying small tumors and strokes, the higher spatial resolution of a structural MRI scan would make it the preferred procedure. Recent developments in insurance and Medicare reimbursement policies, instrumentation, and commercial PET radiopharmaceutical distribution are rapidly making the acquisition of FDG PET scans achievable in routine clinical settings wherever general nuclear medicine services are currently provided. In the past, PET scanners were only available in a limited number of academic centers. However, the recent decision for Medicare reimbursement for the costs of performing PET for some clinical oncology and cardiology indications means that in the future PET is likely to be more widely available in the United States. The Academy of Molecular Imaging reports that 500 PET scanners were in operation in the United States in 2001. Increasingly, low-cost systems and the development of mobile PET services are making this technology more available. The opportunity has thus arrived for making a significant advance in our current approach to evaluating patients for dementia, with use of the tools of molecular-based medical imaging to help elucidate the underlying pathophysiology occurring in the brains of patients who are at an early stage of cognitive decline.

Imaging Embryos to Understand Natal Development

By Wade Roush

In the following selection science journalist Wade Roush describes how advances in medical imaging are enhancing the study of pre-natal development. In the 1980s ultrasound provided the first live-action images of early-stage mammalian fetuses, but clear imaging of embryos had to await further developments. Roush describes how new techniques—including advances in ultrasound, magnetic resonance imaging (MRI), and computer-enhancement of data—are providing the sharpest, most informative images of embryonic development ever. So far, the research has focused largely on mouse embryos that have been removed from the uterus. However, scientists are working on adapting those technologies to capture images of embryos as they develop in the womb. Some researchers are working on techniques to combine images so as to create movies of the embryo's progress. Wade Roush is a senior editor at *Technology Review Magazine.* He holds a doctorate from the Massachusetts Institute of Technology.

For researchers studying how embryos develop, model organisms such as sea urchins, nematodes, and zebra fish have a clear advantage: lucidly transparent embryos that develop outside their mothers' bodies, making it easy to observe their development under a microscope. By contrast, scientists' picture of mammalian embryos, which grow deep in a darkened womb, has long been relatively opaque. Not until the invention of ultrasound imaging in the 1980s did they get their first live—albeit grainy and cryptic—pictures of fetuses romping in the womb. Now, however, mammalian embryology's dark ages may finally be coming to an end.

By adapting established technologies such as ultrasound imaging, confocal microscopy, and magnetic resonance imaging (MRI), researchers are developing new ways to make images of once-hidden embryos. They are also harnessing computers to represent existing molecular data on development in its anatomical context. As a result, they are getting noninvasive views of mouse embryos and preserved human embryos that are sharper, deeper, more dynamic, and—most important—more informative than ever before.

The new technologies are adding a third and a fourth dimension—depth and time—to the two-dimensional (2D) still images found in most scientific reports in embryology. "When we studied [embryogenesis] in school, all we had to look at was a series of tissue sections, and it would take weeks to figure out how they were connected," says developmental biologist Steven Klein of the National Institute of Child Health and Human Development (NICHD) in Bethesda, Maryland. "Here's the chance to take all those sections, reconstruct them into a computer model, and do this for different stages. The result is an interactive movie: You watch it from the front, from the top, and from the side, and you understand development completely."

The Role of Genes

These new imaging capabilities couldn't have come at a better time, developmental biologists say. Over the past decade, advances in molecular biology have allowed researchers to identify many of the genes that drive mammalian embryogenesis. But as Sally Moody, a developmental neurobiologist at the George Washington University Medical Center in Washington, D.C., points out, "Gene function is extremely difficult to ascertain if you don't know the morphology of what's actually going on in the embryo." Now, she says, the high-resolution, three-dimensional (3D) movies of embryogenesis that can be created with the new tools are bringing about "a real melding of genetics and morphology. It's necessary, and it's wonderful."

Moody's comment captures the enthusiasm evident at a developmental imaging workshop held September [1997] at NICHD. Participants said the new techniques can help answer questions they couldn't even ask in the past. How do neural precursor cells fare, for example, when they are transplanted from one spot of the embryonic mouse brain to another? How do subtle malformations in an embryo's cardiac muscles disrupt blood flow through the heart? And how do the membranes and subcellular components of individual cells throb and undulate as the cells migrate to their destined locations?

Beyond such basic-science questions, the meeting even gave a few hints of the eventual practical benefits of the techniques. Physicians at the University of California, San Diego, for example, showed 3D ultrasonograms of fetal faces so clear and lifelike that some pregnant mothers have claimed to see a family resemblance—and have stopped smoking or drinking as a consequence.

Getting to 3-D

The approaches to embryo imaging laid out at the NICHD workshop ranged from the dizzyingly high-tech—for example, miniaturized MRI machines reminiscent of Isaac Asimov's *Fantastic Voyage*—to methods not much more sophisticated than those used to make topographical maps. On the high-tech end, neurobiologist Russell Jacobs and colleagues at the California Institute of Technology in Pasadena are using MRI to add new dimensions to the atlases of development often consulted by researchers and students.

Existing photographic atlases offer 2D images of selected slices of mouse, chick, frog, and other embryos at specific times in development. Jacobs's goal is to produce 3D 2D atlases, then bring in the missing time dimension, stringing together 3D snapshots like an animated cartoon. Magnetic resonance is well-suited to these tasks. Because it uses electromagnetic pulses, rather than harmful x-rays or radioactive dyes, it can be repeatedly applied without damaging an embryo. With the aid of a computer, MR images can then be rendered either as solid, 3D volumes or as 2D cross sections sliced in any direction.

In his first effort, Jacobs has produced MR images of mouse embryos removed from the uterus that are so detailed it's possible to distinguish tissue layers only 50 micrometers thick. But ultimately, Jacobs would like to create such images without removing the embryo from its sanctuary. That's a challenge, he explains, as clinical MRI machines typically produce images with "voxels," or 3D pixels, of about 1 cubic millimeter, but high-resolution images of tiny mouse embryos require voxels 10 million times smaller. When the object is so small relative to an MRI machine's receiver coils, its signal tends to get swamped by background noise, especially if it's surrounded by a lot of other tissue—the mother.

Seeking Live Embryonic Images

But by experimenting with higher magnetic field strengths, different pulse frequencies, and other adjustments to conventional MR imaging machines, Jacobs and his colleagues are gradually increasing signal-to-noise ratios to acceptable levels. "Once you can do [imaging] in vivo, a lot of things open up that are hard to do in vitro," he says. "For one thing, you can follow events over time in the same specimen."

At Duke University Medical Center's Center for In Vivo Microscopy in Durham, North Carolina, researcher Bradley Smith and colleagues are taking a different approach to the noise problem: shrinking the MR receivers down to embryo size, to reduce the size differential between receiver and subject. Smith, who started out as a medical illustrator and then earned a Ph.D. in anatomy so he could "get a peek inside these objects I was drawing," uses the devices to flesh out collaborators' studies of mice or rats with developmental mutations. "They'll perform some manipulation, then turn a pregnant mouse specimen over to me and ask me to investigate the embryos to determine when and where changes are occurring," Smith explains.

Using MR microscopy, for example, Smith has helped researchers compare the vasculature of 12-day-old mouse embryos treated with retinoic acid, a compound that induces birth defects, with normal embryos. The treated embryos lacked blood vessels in their tails and lower limbs, indicating that retinoic acid interferes with developmental signals in the rear half of the embryo.

Right now, getting a high-resolution image requires sacrificing the embryos in order to fix them inside the miniature MR coils. But like Jacobs, Smith says he and other Duke researchers will soon be using the devices to examine live embryos in utero. And in the meantime, other, more serendipitous, uses for the technology are emerging.

One came from a team of physicists, who asked Smith's help in working out how much radiation human embryos are likely to absorb when, for example, female nuclear workers or scientists using radioactive chemicals are exposed before realizing they are pregnant. The physicists needed data about the size and volume of embryonic organs at different times in development in order to estimate how much of the radiation reaching the womb an embryo would actually absorb. Smith provided this data by doing MR studies of the human embryos in the historical Carnegie Collection at the Armed Forces Institute of Pathology in Washington, D.C., and then deriving 3D images of the embryos.

Tracing Primitive Brain Cells

At the Skirball Institute of Biomolecular Medicine at New York University School of Medicine in Manhattan, developmental neurobiologist Dan Turnbull is adapting another established imaging technique to carry out delicate microsurgical procedures on mouse embryos still in the womb. Turnbull studies the transformation of ectodermal tissue into brain cells in the mouse embryo. To learn exactly when neural progenitor cells in different regions of the primordial mouse brain become committed to their ultimate fates, he and co-workers Martin Olsson and Kenneth Campbell are using high-frequency, high-resolution ultrasound imaging to guide the needles used in cell transplantation experiments.

When the researchers grafted marked cells from the forebrains of 13-day-old mouse embryos to specific spots in mid-hindbrain and vice versa, they reported in the October issue of *Neuron*, they found that the dislocated forebrain cells metamorphosed into hindbrain cells, while the grafted hindbrain cells failed to adapt to their new location—indicating that the fates of hindbrain cells are set before those of forebrain cells.

Just as important as this result was the precedent set by the experiment. Such cell transplants had never before been attempted on such young mouse embryos. But the technique allowed the researchers to distinguish the tiny structures—the entire embryonic mouse brain at that stage is only a few millimeters thick—sufficiently well to perform the transplants. "A lot of people who have come to our institute and seen us doing these procedures have been getting excited," says Turnbull. "Everybody sees the future applications where we can start introducing labeled cells into mutant mice, to look at how the differentiation process is altered."

Making 3-D Movies

Perhaps the greatest excitement at the NICHD workshop, however, was sparked by another effort to image individual cells. Researchers at the University of Iowa's W. M. Keck Dynamic Image Analysis Facility in Iowa City have melded a confocal microscope[1] a 3D movie camera and a computer to create the world's only instrument for monitoring the full range of movements and shape changes that cells undergo during development. The microscope changes its focal plane 30 times per second, and the computer records the resulting "optical sections" for reconstruction into a 3D computer model that highlights cell membranes and internal surfaces such as those of the nucleus, mitochondria, and vesicles. The process is repeated every 2 seconds, and a Quick-Time movie is the result.

So far, the technique has been used only on cells that can crawl in a lab dish. David Soll, director of the Keck facility, handed out red-and-blue glasses at the workshop and treated viewers to a 3D movie of the sluglike colonies that the normally unicellular slime mold Dictyostelium forms when it needs to reproduce. Like all amoeboid creatures, the Dictyostelium colony moves by continuously assembling and disassembling its internal skeleton, made of the protein actin. Soll's movie showed how the colonies pulsate as their actin-filled pseudopods appear and disappear, dragging along the entire mass.

Using the 3D motion analysis system, Soll and his collaborators have demonstrated that Dictyostelium strains engineered to lack certain of the proteins known to regulate actin display specific flaws in the way they create or absorb pseudopods. These flaws are a sign that the numerous cytoskeletal regulators aren't redundant, but specialized. According to George Washington's Moody, that result would probably elude a researcher viewing mutant Dictyostelium colonies under a conventional 2D microscope.

And that in the end, may be the strongest rationale behind the

1. a laser-aided narrow-focus microscope that permits ultrahigh-resolution images of extremely small areas of interest, which can be combined to form larger, detailed images

new surge in developmental imaging. Reseachers using 2D still images of their subjects have to spend years acquiring an ethereal, intuitive "feeling for the organism" before they can understand its behavior in three dimensions over time, Moody argues. "But having these new technologies out there means that people will quickly be able to form a visual understanding they can rely on. . . . Its going to be terrific."

Functional MRI Reveals the Brain at Work

By Marcia Barinaga

The human brain is composed of soft tissues encased in hard bone. That structural arrangement has made imaging this most complex of all biological organs a challenge. In the following selection science writer Marcia Barinaga describes how advances in imaging technologies have allowed researchers to see the brain in action for the first time. The key to progress has been the development of functional magnetic resonance imaging, or fMRI. This technique tracks the flow of blood to various centers of the brain, Barinaga explains. Since active parts of the brain require more oxygen than inactive ones, the blood flow images present a portrait of brain activity.

Scientists are working on many fronts to develop additional techniques to extract more detail from brain imaging. Barinaga reports that Harvard researchers have developed computer analysis techniques that have reduced the waiting time between fMRI brain scans from sixteen seconds to just two. Other scientists have produced images of a small area of the brain so rapidly that they can be strung together to make a movie. Still others have combined fMRI with techniques that more sensitively measure the timing of events in the brain.

Looking ahead, Barinaga says researchers are currently attempting to find ways to use fMRI to measure brain activity not from blood flow but directly from the changes in neurons themselves. Some other researchers are looking into alternative imaging technologies. Optical imaging, which involves shining a light at bone-penetrating wavelengths through the skull, may eventually supplement fMRI, she reports. Marcia Barinaga, a contributing correspondent to

Marcia Barinaga, "New Imaging Methods Provide a Better View into the Brain," *Science,* vol. 276, June 27, 1997, p. 1,974. Copyright © 1997 by the American Association for the Advancement of Science. Reproduced by permission.

Science, writes primarily about neuroscience. She is based in the magazine's bureau in Berkeley, California.

For a field that didn't even exist 20 years ago, human brain imaging has developed at a mind-boggling pace. Thanks to one advance after another, neurobiologists can peer into the living human brain and produce pictures that shed new light on brain functions ranging from the processing of sensory information to higher level thinking tasks. But breathtaking as the developments have been, improvements already under way will soon give imagers new perspectives on how the brain goes about its business.

Most of these advances are based on functional magnetic resonance imaging (fMRI), a technique that spots the increases in the blood oxygenation that reflect a boost in blood flow to active brain areas. Because of advantages—including greater speed and higher resolution—in recent years, fMRI has largely eclipsed positron emission tomography (PET), the method that got the imaging field rolling nearly 20 years ago. Now, researchers are devising a whole new wave of modifications, several of which were showcased at a recent conference on brain imaging, that will allow fMRI to be used to even better advantage.

Some modifications will permit more sophisticated experimental designs that link brain images more closely to a subject's perceptions and behavior. In addition, increased magnet strengths will give even greater spatial resolution of activated brain areas. By combining fMRI with other techniques, researchers are now able to answer previously unaddressable questions about the timing with which brain areas are activated. Those answers will yield insights into how information moves through the brain.

More to Come

As these advances invigorate the field, a next wave is waiting in the wings: methods that may image neural activity directly by following the flux of sodium ions, or by measuring the scattering of light by brain tissue. These newest directions are as yet unproven, but in a field where methods go from inconceivable to commonplace in a couple of years, researchers have learned never to say never. "I hesitate to say [any technique] isn't going anywhere, because I could be writing a grant to try to buy the equipment in 2 years," jokes cognitive neuroscientist George Mangun of the University of California (UC), Davis.

Mangun learned that lesson, he says, from the fast ascent of fMRI. When he heard of an early form of the technique in 1990, Mangun recalls, he thought the technique was "interesting . . . but [would] never go anywhere." Within a year, additional advances had paved the way for it to become the mainstay of the field.

But even as fMRI was catapulting to its position of prominence, researchers using the technique unwittingly handicapped themselves with old habits carried over from PET imaging that have prevented them from taking full advantage of fMRI. PET, which uses radioactive tracers to detect the increased blood flow to activated brain regions, is slow, taking up to a minute to gather the data for a brain image. As a result, neuroscientists using the method do "block trials," in which the subject performs a string of similar short tasks, causing the brain to repeat the same mental process while the data are gathered. Researchers continued to use block trials with fMRI, although that technique takes only 2 seconds to collect an image. "We always assumed if we only looked at one trial, the signal would be so small we wouldn't be able to see it," says neuroimager Randy Buckner of Harvard Medical School in Boston.

That assumption evaporated in 1995, when Robert Savoy and his colleagues at Harvard Medical School reported that fMRI could detect brain activations in response to a visual stimulus lasting only 30 milliseconds. The next year, Buckner and his colleagues did a similar experiment with a cognitive task. They used the word-stem completion test, in which subjects are given three-letter parts of words and asked to complete the word. A single word-stem completion, the researchers found, activated brain areas nearly identical to those activated by a block trial.

Thus was born a new method, "event-related" fMRI, in which researchers collect brain image data from individual trials, which they can then sort and pool as they wish. It opens up many avenues for cognitive experiments, says Buckner. For example, some tests don't work well in block trials, because they involve an element of surprise.

Mapping Brain Activity

Studies with electroencephalograms (EEGs), which record electrical activity inside the brain, have demonstrated that if you show a person a series of pictures, say, of geometric shapes, and then throw in something different, like a picture of an animal, the oddball picture produces a bigger neural response than the others. Neuroimagers would like to know which brain areas react to the surprise, but they can't find out from a block experiment, says Buckner, because "if you do that kind of surprise three or four times, [the response] goes away." With event-related fMRI, researchers can mix "surprise" trials with other types of trials, and then afterward pool the data from the surprise trials to analyze together.

Research groups have leaped to use the new approach, not only to identify brain areas that react to unusual events, but also to relate brain activity directly to subjects' responses or perceptions which can only be determined once the experimental trial is over. For example, the technique allows researchers to sort brain images based on whether a subject got the right or wrong answer in a test, and see how the brain activation differed. Because of its ability to address some of these important questions with imaging for the first time, the technique "is catching on incredibly rapidly," says Buckner.

It is likely to catch on even faster, thanks to some recent troubleshooting done by Buckner and his Harvard colleague Anders Dale. The problem they addressed is this: The fMRI response to a single trial takes more than 10 seconds to run its course, so it seemed that individual trials would have to be separated by 16 seconds or so to be sure the response to one trial was finished before the next one was presented. That is not only time-consuming, but could also alter the results. "Sixteen seconds is a long time to do nothing," says Buckner. "People have more time to work on the problem, more time to prepare." Dale and Buckner have a paper in press in Human Brain Mapping showing that trials can be presented as fast as every 2 seconds, and an algorithm can then be used to extract the overlapping brain activation data associated with each trial.

Ever-More Powerful Magnets

Advances like event-related fMRI have opened up countless questions for cognitive neuroscientists to address. Most can be tackled using standard fMRI machines, which have magnetic field strengths of 1.5 or 3 teslas (T) and can distinguish activated brain areas separated by as little as half a centimeter. But "there will be a time when we will definitely have to look beyond" that resolution, says brain imager Kamil Ugurbil of the University of Minnesota, Minneapolis. Ugurbil, who feels that time is rapidly approaching, is leading the charge to higher magnetic fields. The imaging center at Minnesota has a 4-T MRI machine, one of only a handful in the world. With those machines, researchers have revealed multiple strengths of higher fields.

At higher fields, Ugurbil says, event-related fMRI can be developed to its full potential, producing robust images from single trials, and reducing the need for researchers to sort and pool their results. What's more, researchers have already seen two brain features with 4-T machines that have eluded those using lesser magnetic fields. One, the so-called early oxygenation dip, is an apparent drop in blood oxygenation in active brain areas before the rise in blood flow (*Science*, 11 April, p. 196). Researchers using 4 T have also seen ocular dominance columns—columns of neurons in the visual cortex with diameters on the order of 1 millimeter—which respond selectively to images from one eye or the other. All these effects are sure to be even clearer at fields higher than 4 T, Ugurbil says.

Indeed, neuroimager Roger Tootell, of Harvard Medical School in Boston, calls Ugurbil's sighting of ocular dominance columns a "watershed" in brain imaging. Imagers now focus on activity in whole brain areas, but the opportunity to see the activity of individual columns within those areas promises "a quantum jump in insight," Tootell says. "There are columns all over the brain, and we don't know what they do."

Ugurbil's team hopes to pursue both the oxygenation dip and column resolution with a 7-T human imaging machine they are due to receive in December. It will be the first of its kind in the world. But no human has ever been exposed to a 7-T field, and safety tests on animals, already begun by Ugurbil's group, will be needed before that can be done.

Even if those colossal fields are deemed safe, neuroimager Marcus Raichle of Washington University in St. Louis warns that bigger is not better for everyone, because the bigger machines require an engineering team devoted to tinkering and tuning constantly. "You become hostage to the equipment if you're not careful," he says, likening a high-field magnet to a "Ferrari that needs a $5000 tune-up every year" and isn't really suited to just going for a ride. "A well-equipped, well-running 1.5-T machine, with . . . people who know how to ask the questions, is an enormously powerful piece of equipment," Raichle argues. "There is a tremendous amount of neurobiology that can and will be done on such machines." Nevertheless, he says, someone, preferably with Ugurbil's level of experience, needs to be developing higher field machines to pave the way for a time when the biological questions demand the next wave in resolution. "We may, 5 years from now, say, 'Gosh, we all have to be at 5 T.'"

A Timely Union

One trick not even the biggest MRI machine can presently pull off on its own is following precisely when brain areas become active during a cognitive process. That's because the neurons themselves respond within 10 milliseconds of a triggering stimulus, while the blood-flow changes measured by fMRI or PET take several seconds to develop. This limitation has been a great frustration for neuroimagers. "Timing is everything in the brain," says UC Davis's Mangun. Without timing information, researchers can only guess about how different brain areas build on each other's work as they perform a task.

To remedy this problem, Mangun's group and others have recently arranged a marriage of convenience between fMRI and PET imaging techniques and a pair of brain-recording methods whose forte is timing: EEG, which measures the electrical fields produced by brain neuron activity, and magnetoencephalography (MEG), which measures neurally generated magnetic fields. Both methods can take readings at more than 100 points on the scalp and can track how neural activity changes with time along the surface of the head. But they have a big weakness: They can't pinpoint the source of the electromagnetic signal.

Mathematical equations can point to brain areas where the activity might be, but the equations yield multiple solutions, with no way to tell which one is right. But "if you can calculate a [candidate] position, and then show that neuroimaging shows that there are active cells in that particular place, then that increases your confidence that you've got it right," says EEG researcher Steven Hillyard of UC San Diego.

Locating the Attention Center

Hans-Jochen Heinze at Otto von Guericke University in Magdeburg, Germany, along with Mangun and Hillyard, did just that with a cognitive task in 1994. They presented subjects with pairs of symbols in both their right and left visual fields and directed their attention to either the right or left field by asking them to judge whether the symbols appearing there were the same or different. Earlier work in Hillyard's lab had shown that the EEG wave evoked by the symbols differs, depending on whether the subject is paying attention to them or not: A bump in the wave beginning about 80 milliseconds after the symbols were flashed, known as the P1 component, gets bigger when the subject pays attention.

To find the source of the activity that creates P1, the Heinze team had the subjects do the task once while the researchers took EEG recordings, and again in the PET scanner. The PET data showed two areas in the so-called "extrastriate" portion of the visual cortex that could be the source of P1, and the team then returned to the model to see whether these spots would work as possible sources that would explain the EEG data. Those sites, says Mangun, explained the data "very, very well." Mangun has since shown that making the perceptual task easier selectively reduces both P1 and the attention-associated extrastriate activation seen in PET, further support that the two techniques are measuring the same brain function.

That experiment showed that imaging and electromagnetic techniques can work together, says Harvard's Dale. But the math used by the Heinze team could consider only two or three simultaneously active brain areas as possible sources of the EEG signal. And while that was fine in the case they had chosen, Dale points out that in most cognitive processes, many brain areas are activated. Dale is one of several researchers deriving a new generation of mathematical models that can pose thousands of sites of brain activity as potential sources and contain other improvements as well.

Like the model used by the Heinze group, Dale's model begins with electromagnetic data recorded on the scalp and predicts which configuration of active areas in the brain could best explain that activity. But instead of relying just on EEG recordings, it can use MEG and EEG data taken simultaneously. And while older methods model the brain as a sphere inside the skull, Dale's limits the potential sources of activity to the cerebral cortex. Moreover, because each brain is unique in how its cortex is folded, Dale uses a structural MR image to tailor the calculations to the individual brain.

The result is a localized, though fuzzy, estimate of combined activity in the brain that could produce the EEG and MEG signals at any point in time. Dale then takes fMRI data on brain activity during an identical experimental trial and uses those data to "weight" the solutions by having the equations favor areas shown to be active by the fMRl. The end result is a set of crisp images with the spatial resolution of fMRI that show changes in brain activity on a time scale of tens of milliseconds. "You can make a movie animating this," Dale says.

Dale, Tootell, and Jack Belliveau, also of Harvard, have validated the technique by using it to look at the timing of the brain's response to a moving image, and Dale and Eric Halgren of UC Los Angeles have studied the time course with which the brain responds to novel versus repeated words. "It is an important wedding of techniques," says Washington University's Raichle and is likely to become a staple of the field for researchers who want to know the pathways information takes in the course of a thinking process.

Working with Sodium

Millisecond movies of neural activity using fMRI, EEG, and MEG might seem visionary enough, but some in the field think such wonders will someday be possible with a single technique— either a new form of fMRI or a much less expensive alternative: imaging with ordinary light beams.

Keith Thulborn's team at the University of Pittsburgh Medical Center is working to devise a way to get images with real-time resolution information directly from fMRI, by measuring changes in the sodium magnetic resonance signal. "Sodium imaging may be a very direct way of looking at neuronal activity," says Thulborn, because sodium ions flow into neurons when they fire. The passage of ions into the neurons changes sodium's magnetic resonance properties in a way that should be detectable by MRI, Thulborn says.

The imaging center at Pittsburgh already uses sodium imaging clinically to assess brain damage in patients with strokes, epilepsy, and tumors. Because the sodium signals are weak, it takes 10 minutes to create a reliable three-dimensional image, says Thulborn. But because MR images are built up from many individual snapshots, Thulborn says it would be possible to construct images that capture the immediate neural response by taking repeated snapshots timed at a very short interval after a repeated stimulus. Thulborn and a team of engineers and physicists have been working for 6 years to improve the MRI machine's ability to detect sodium. Their work has reduced the detection time from 45 minutes to 10, while increasing spatial resolution an order of magnitude, and they plan to test the experimental approach on a 3-T machine within the next few months.

Using Light to Get Images

Still other researchers are hoping to image neural activity directly without the $1-million-per-tesla price tag of fMRI. Their preferred medium: light. Studies in living brain slices have shown that the light-scattering properties of neurons change when they become active. Cognitive neuroscientists Gabriele Gratton and Monica Fabiani of the University of Missouri, Columbia, lead one of several labs trying to take advantage of that property by using near-infrared light from a fiber-optic source to image activity changes in living human brains. Their system, which they call EROS, for event-related optical signals, has a bargain-basement cost of less than $50,000.

When a fiber-optic source placed on the scalp shines light into the head, the light penetrates the skull and is scattered by brain tissues before some of it reemerges. EROS uses light sensors placed on the scalp just centimeters from the source to measure the time the light takes to emerge. Because that time is influenced by light scattering, which in turn is affected by neural activity, the system can detect changes induced by an experimental task. And it does it with a temporal resolution similar to that of an EEG. EROS can also locate the source of the scattering changes, based on detector placement and timing of the light's emergence, with spatial resolution of less than a centimeter. Using EROS, Gratton repeated the experiment by which Heinze, Mangun, and Hillyard first showed the power of combining PET with EEG. EROS produced the same results, localizing the effects of attention to the extrastriate cortex.

One limitation of EROS is that the light can only penetrate several centimeters into the head, and so the technique is unable to register activity from deep brain areas. Indeed, some researchers worry that it will not reliably image parts of the cortex that are buried in folds. "If it is limited to the superficial cortex, it will never replace fMRI," says cognitive neuroscientist Steven Luck, of the University of Iowa, Iowa City. But Gratton and Fabiani say they have already imaged cortical areas deep in a fold and have ideas about how to reach even deeper regions.

"My eye is on optical techniques in terms of the next wave," says neuroimager Bruce Rosen, of the magnetic resonance imaging center at Harvard Medical School. "In 10 years, I wonder if we will all be doing optical imaging and throwing away our magnets." While most brain imagers might think that unlikely, this is a field that has learned never to say never.

Laser Imaging May Improve Mammography

By Laurie Toupin

Mammography, the imaging of breasts to search for incipient cancer, has traditionally been performed by X-rays. The procedure, which involves pressing the breasts as flat as possible to spread out the tissues, is uncomfortable and sometimes painful. In the following selection science writer Laurie Toupin describes new mammography technology that avoids the need for breast compression and bypasses X-rays altogether. The Computer Tomography Laser Mammography system relies on an infrared laser that rotates around the breast to obtain a series of scans that eventually maps the entire breast. As the laser shines, detectors record both the absorption and emission of light from the breast. A combination of the two images allows a diagnostician to pinpoint any suspicious tissues. The system offers a potential for treatment as well, Toupin reports. A glowing "biochemical fluorescence tag" could be used to mark a tumor, she writes, and then light from the laser could be used to activate drugs to kill it.

The Computer Tomography Laser Mammography system has undergone a series of clinical tests to determine its safety and effectiveness. As of late 2004, Imaging Diagnostics Systems, Inc., the company that makes the device, was working to get U.S. Food and Drug Administration approval to market it. Laurie Toupin is a freelance science writer for children and adults. She writes from her home in Pepperell, Massachusetts.

Physicians and women patients alike will appreciate the Computer Tomography Laser Mammography (CTLM Trademark) breast-imaging system from Imaging Diagnostics

Systems Inc. (IDSI). The reason: Not only does the instrument perform comfortable, non-invasive detection, but it potentially will be able to treat cancer as well, saving time.

To obtain a 3D image of the breast and its internal structures, a patient lies face down on the scanning bed. Her breast hangs free into a well in the bed called the scanning chamber. An infrared laser, emitted on a horizontal plane, rotates 360 degrees. The computer acquires data at one horizontal level "slice," then lowers the detectors and laser, typically 4 mm, to image another section.

A specially designed double-row detector array images both the absorption and florescence of breast tissue. The optical mammography system maps local changes in the optical scattering and absorption coefficients over the cross sections. When the absorption and fluorescence images are overlaid, a diagnostician can determine the exact location of any problem. "To the best of our knowledge, this is the first time this type of imaging has been done anywhere in the world," says Richard Grable, IDSI CEO.

Potential for Use in Treatment

Because the scanner images fluorescence, a surgeon potentially can use a biochemical fluorescence tag to locate the tumor and then turn around and use the same device to treat the disease through photodynamic therapy. In photodynamic therapy, specially developed photoresponsive drugs administered to the patient preferentially locate within cancerous tissue. When the compounds are illuminated by light at the activating wavelength, they release singlet oxygen that immediately kills the adjacent cells.

After five years in development, the instrument debuted in July 1999. But after its first clinical test, "We quickly saw that the real world environment of the hospital was quite hostile compared to our lab," says Grable. Not only did the quickly varying temperature in a hospital room create instabilities in the laser system, but also the size of the instrument was unwieldy.

So IDSI engineers went from a four-laser system down to one and reduced the size of the instrument by 45% in only 10 working days. This quick turn-around time was the result of fortuitous engineering from the start, says Grable. The scanner was designed so that one could change the detector or electronics without having a huge impact on the mechanical parts.

Realizing they may have had the answer in an older design, engineers "went back to the bone yard and pulled parts from a system that we developed a couple of years ago," says Robert Wake, IDSI director of engineering. "Manufacturing resurrected the instrument and engineering designed a way to incorporate the new laser diode."

The mechanical framework, the rotation and lift mechanism, and the fiberglass skins haven't changed for three years, says Wake, "yet we've made several different scanners. We're pleased with how much mileage we've gotten out of the original design."

Two diode-pumped solid-state lasers, one Ti-sapphire laser, and one regenerative amplifier were replaced with one diode laser and a proprietary controller for temperature and power.

Also, the 85 200-micron glass-fiber optic cables originally used to transmit captured light to the detector electronics were eliminated through a new detection layout. The first instrument performed at only 60% efficiency. "We were throwing away 40% of our light," says Grable. "This is fine if you are working with a powerful output, but we were losing part of the signal we were trying to detect." Engineers solved the problem by positioning the large area photo diodes closer to the breast, reducing the need for so many fiber-optic cables.

Increased Efficiency

Between the move to one laser and the new detection design, engineers were able to eliminate many of the special optical amplifiers, says Grable. "All we have now is a single console with the computer, a 21-inch monitor, keyboard, and the scanning bed where the patient lies down."

Along with the decreased size and decreased cost of lasers came increased reliability. "Reliability is a big thing in hospitals. Down time doesn't help patients. The way the lasers were before, we didn't have the uptime we needed to get the throughput," Grable adds.

The scanner's high-gloss "automotive finish" is also unique for an instrument this size, says Grable. "A crackle finish hides a lot of sins. But we didn't want to go that route." So IDSI hired a design company to create an attractive physical appearance. But maintaining this high-quality finish while developing a precise mold became a challenge.

IDSI engineers originally drew the design in AutoCAD from

Autodesk (San Rafael, CA). They later migrated the data to Solid-Works (Concord, MA). "We used stereo lithography to make tenth-scale models," says Wake. To create the fiberglass molds, engineers made a male part by cutting laminated cardboard sheets directly from CAD files, from which they made the female molds.

All the parts were designed on the computer, says Wake. Not one physical drawing was involved. "There is no other easy way to do this because all the compound curves would be difficult to draw and dimension," says Wake. "Ironically, our Q/A people are now asking for drawings so they can inspect the parts in production. We have to go back and generate them.". . .

It has been a real learning curve, says Grable. "We use the analogy that it's like peeling an onion. You peel back one layer only to find another. It's taken awhile to get to the center." The design continually evolves.

"From the start, we wanted to be confident that the design would survive the life span of the machine with virtually no maintenance of the mechanical parts," says Wake. So IDSI performed a one-million-slice life-cycle test on the fiber cable system and related mechanical parts including the drive chain, the mechanism for raising and lowering the platform, and the motor that rotated the lasers.

"We had to know if we were building a monster or not," says Grable.

Tests Under Way

And since none of the fiber optic venders knew if their product could survive such a test, "We bit the bullet and tested for 24 hours a day, 7 days a week, for six months," Wake says. IDSI engineers illuminated the fibers at one end and, once a day, took a frame grab video picture of the other end to ensure there was no leakage from micro fractures or broken fibers. "We were also careful never to violate the bend radius of the fibers, making sure the cable swept a very generous arc inside the machine," he added. And the results: no degradation whatsoever.

Although not quite ready for prime time, two clinical studies are currently under way [in 2000] at the University of Virginia and Nassau County, NY medical centers. Grable hopes to have some version of their scanner marketable by Thanksgiving [2000].

Computers Are Vital to New Imaging Techniques

By Anthony Brinton Wolbarst

Computers have entered into nearly every aspect of medical imaging. In the following selection physicist Anthony Brinton Wolbarst considers how digital images are formed and what advantages they confer to those working in the medical imaging field. Digital images offer many advantages, he states. Images can be enhanced pixel by pixel to bring out details. The images can then be transmitted almost instantaneously great distances via phone lines or the Internet. Computers also allow traditional X-ray images to be enlarged or rotated. More important, when employed in computed tomography and magnetic resonance procedures, computers make it possible to create highly detailed three-dimensional images of internal organs. Moreover, computers are opening the way for doctors to take virtual-reality tours inside their patients, and even to rehearse a surgical procedure before actually performing it. The role of computers in medical imaging, Wolbarst writes, is bound to grow. Anthony Wolbarst is program director of the Division of Applied Science and Technology at the National Institutes of Health. He holds a doctorate in physics and has served on the faculty of Harvard Medical School and on the staff of the National Cancer Institute.

Anthony Brinton Wolbarst, *Looking Within: How X-Ray, CT, MRI, Ultrasound, and Other Medical Images Are Created, and How They Help Physicians Save Lives.* Berkeley: University of California Press, 1999. Copyright © 1999 by The Regents of the University of California. Reproduced by permission.

How does an image get into a computer in the first place? The name of the game is digitization, and in its simplest form, digitizing an image is just the converse of painting by numbers.

Suppose we want to modify that famous old World War I black and white photograph of Bill Garrison [an elderly patient] in his Sopwith Camel, and show him landing next to a 747. We install all the necessary art and design software into a PC, and attach some sort of electronic image acquisition device, such as a scanner or a CCD [charge-coupled device; i.e., digital] camera, and point it at the photo. The system starts off by partitioning the image into an imaginary mosaic of many very small picture elements, or *pixels*, each with a unique numerical *pixel address* that indicates its spatial location. . . . The optical input device and computer would chop the image into an array of adjacent squares, in effect, and then number them sequentially in a raster pattern [rows of pixels]—like numbering the positions of the characters and spaces as you read from this page. Our photo-imaging unit then views and measures the degree of darkness in each pixel, and translates it into a numerical *pixel value.* The entire image can thus be represented and stored in memory as a long listing of pairs of numbers: the pixel addresses and corresponding pixel values. Now we're ready to use a graphics program to play with the image—in this case, excising the biplane and inserting it into a digitized shot of JFK Airport.

Digitizing an X-Ray Image

Digitizing a radiographic film is done essentially the same way. Let's say a surgeon in San Diego needs to study a patient's film taken and archived last month in New York City—and she needs it right away. Once the required radiograph is located (which could take considerable time, since it's buried in a stack of films in Dr. Jones's office, and he's off on a month-long lecture and golf tour of Burkina Faso), it is entered into a digitizer. . . . There, within a light-proof box, the film lies flat on a horizontal glass plate. A laser points at it from above, and a computer-controlled mechanical or electro-optical device deflects and aims the narrow laser beam to successive points on the film. The amount of laser light that gets through any small area of the film is continuously monitored by a photodetector beneath the glass plate.

To begin digitization, the computer partitions the film into an imaginary matrix of square picture elements—whose dimensions are roughly those of the laser beam itself—and assigns a spatial address to each. It then directs the laser beam to the first of these pixels, and the photodetector generates a voltage proportional to the amount of laser light transmitted through that tiny area of film. The signal voltage from the photodetector is measured and electronically digitized—transformed into an ordinary number, expressed in bits and bytes. This number is sent back to the computer, which now knows both the position and the amount of darkening of this small portion of film. The laser beam then proceeds rapidly to the next pixel location, and the photodetector samples the film transparency there, too, and generates the corresponding pixel value, and so on. The two-dimensional matrix of numbers produced in this fashion is called a "bit map." The computer can store—or send to California electronically—the bit map as a long string of pixel addresses and values.

Once in the computer, and perhaps after some digital enhancement, the image can be made to reappear on a display by reversing the digitization process. The computer pulls up all the stored pixel addresses and pixel values for a single image, and places them in proper sequence according to the raster pattern. The digital numeric address of the first pixel is converted into voltages that, for a television monitor, deflect its electron beam so that the point of light on the screen moves to the correct pixel location; the pixel value controls the display brightness (and perhaps color) there. Then on to the second pixel. This happens extraordinarily quickly, of course, but the individual steps are straightforward.

For the film digitizer, the laser-plus-photodetector system scanned a radiograph and generated a signal voltage that was then digitized and sent to a computer. . . . Other digital imaging systems work much the same way. The types of radiation that interact with the patient's body and then with the detector(s) differ considerably among different imaging modalities, but for all cases the process is basically the same: a detector senses radiation coming from or modified by the body, and produces a corresponding signal voltage. This electrical signal is digitized and sent to a computer, which produces two- or three-dimensional images that reflect the characteristics of the tissues within the region being examined.

Some information is inevitably lost in sampling and digitizing and re-displaying, so the system must be designed to ensure that the image is not so badly degraded that it is no longer useful. . . . Nothing smaller than a pixel can be imaged, so fine features will be missed if the pixels are too large relative to the entity being viewed, and too small in number. . . . Likewise, even with good resolution, the image will not convey sufficient information unless there are enough distinct gray levels available. And even with an adequate pixel matrix and gray scale, the image will appear over- or underexposed unless the levels of gray are set so as to span and reflect the proper range for the tissue characteristic being imaged.

With a matrix two thousand pixels on a side, a digital radiographic image is nearly indistinguishable from an ordinary X-ray film. CT and MRI enjoy less inherent spatial resolution, by comparison, and often there is little harm in adopting a coarser pixel matrix, such as 512×512, to cover roughly the same region of the body. Nuclear medicine and ultrasound generally require even less fineness. Fewer pixels (or gray levels) per image means faster image reconstruction and processing, and lower storage and communication costs. Thus, an important objective in designing or purchasing imaging equipment is to create an overall system with more than enough capability to accomplish the requisite clinical tasks, but not much beyond that, to keep the cost down.

Direct to Digital

I have described how an ordinary X-ray film can be optically scanned for input into a computer. Digital radiology is a technology in which planar X-ray images are obtained without ever being placed on film—a great leap beyond film digitization.

With one common form of digital radiography, an *imaging plate* coated with a photosensitive phosphor replaces the film-screen cassette as the image receptor. After a normal X-ray exposure, the imaging plate is not developed chemically, like a film. Instead, it is placed inside a light-tight box, and a laser beam of one color of light scans it in a raster pattern while a photodetector continuously monitors how much fluorescent light of a different color is emitted. The brightness of the stimulated light coming from any point on the plate is proportional to the amount of X-ray energy that has passed through the patient and been deposited there. The X-ray image is recovered in the form of the time-varying voltage from the photodetector, somewhat like that from the target of a video camera, and entered into a computer.

Digital radiography offers several benefits. With conventional film X rays, the film has to play two distinct and separate roles. First, it acquires the image: then, after it is developed, it serves as the means of storing and displaying the image. The problem is that exposure conditions that create strong shadows and excellent contrast in the (invisible) X-ray beam emerging from the patient's body are not necessarily the same as those that produce high visual quality in the developed film. Exposure conditions that yield strongest X-ray contrast might make areas of the developed film too faint or too dark to be seen clearly—and once a film has been over- or underexposed, little can be done to fix it.

Digital radiography, on the other hand, permits nearly complete decoupling of image formation from image display, so that each can be optimized separately. That is, first the X-ray machine exposure is set at values that give rise to the greatest differences in attenuation of the beam by the various tissues; afterward, and independently, the operator can manipulate the gray scale, activate contrast-enhancement programs or noise-reduction filters, and adjust other display parameters to obtain the most visually effective image. This flexibility, along with the general advantages of storing and communicating images digitally from the outset, suggest that despite its greater cost, digital radiography will replace film in many situations. The computer's ability to enhance image contrast and to draw a physician's attention to abnormal image patterns may prove particularly useful where irregularities are most subtle, as in mammography. . . .

Major Roles of Computers

Computers play crucial roles in medicine, and nowhere more prominently than in imaging. Although film radiography is still the most common form of imaging, radiologists and other physicians rely more and more on information from computer-based technologies—for several different but interrelated reasons.

Image Reconstruction

Computers, and the digital representation of images, are essential for CT [computed tomography], MRI [magnetic resonance imaging], and PET [positron emission tomography]. These types of images are not obtained directly, as with X-ray film, but are mathematically constructed out of thousands of separate measurements. Without the ability to orchestrate these measurements and then to manipulate their results numerically, performing millions of computations in a few seconds, such imaging simply would not be possible.

Image Processing

Once it's in digital form, any image can be mathematically massaged to improve its appearance and usefulness. Parts or all of it can be enlarged or reduced, rotated, inverted, stretched, or transformed from a positive image to a negative. The computer can adjust the gray scale, which relates pixel value to brightness, to optimize apparent contrast. It can draw a sharp edge where the shade of gray changes abruptly, so as to increase artificially the sharpness of a border, and thus help the eye to distinguish clinically relevant patterns. Digital filters can reduce some kinds of visual noise, compensate for certain inherent inadequacies of the imaging system, and in other ways improve perceived image quality. Such image processing can make the difference between a clinical study that is definitive and one that contributes nothing. . . .

Image Display

Computers make possible various new kinds of display for images, a flexibility that can enhance both their aesthetic appeal and their clinical usefulness. For example, nuclear medicine and ultrasound commonly use "false colors" that indicate places where interesting things are going on. A PET scan might show areas of unusually high uptake of radionuclide in red, and cooler areas with blue; that may (or may not) be diagnostically helpful. Likewise, some special display programs allow different technologies such as MRI and PET to combine dissimilar kinds of information in a single composite image—a situation in which the diagnostic value of the whole may exceed that of the sum of the parts.

With volume-imaging modalities, such as multislice CT, MRI, and PET, regions of concern can be shown either in the form of single slices, as in conventional CT, or in three dimensions. The three-dimensional rendering of organs and bones can assist in preoperative planning for neuro-, facial, and orthopedic surgery, and in the planning of radiotherapy cancer treatment. . . .

One possible next step beyond a three-dimensional image display of a skull is a three-dimensional plastic replication of it. From multislice CT or MRI information, a "fabricator" can generate such an object, one thin layer at a time, from a liquid polymer that hardens when exposed to laser light. Automatic stacking and fusing together of the resulting shaped, solid thin slices can yield a life- (or any other) size model skull that the physician can actually hold—a nearly exact copy of the real thing! (You may have created animals in a similar fashion as a child, gluing together shaped layers of cardboard.)

Exploring Virtual Reality

Virtual reality interactive display systems provide an alternative to solid replications of organs and bones. Virtual endoscopy allows the physician to move around within a three-dimensional block of anatomy, in effect, viewing areas in it from any desired vantage point—along the colon, for example, or down the air pathways. Until recently the stuff of science fiction, such display systems are coming to play important roles in the planning of surgical cases. They would allow surgeons to employ virtual scalpels to peel away and repair virtual tissue and bone, before actually performing the operation, all the while observing the changes as they occur, and undoing them as needed.

Image Archiving and Communications

When in digital form, images from every diagnostic device in a medical center can be entered into a shared computer data base. Any study can be stored inexpensively or retrieved almost instantaneously at every work station, integrated with other kinds of information (such as lab reports, electrocardiogram tracings, general medical records, or perhaps even other images), and transmitted through the hospital or across the continent in seconds. Likewise, through *teleradiology*, a digital image produced at an isolated clinic or hospital can be sent by phone or a dedicated channel to a major medical center for examination by specialists. . . . With powerful image archiving and communications capabilities, physicians can obtain and exchange critical information in minutes, rather than days or weeks, and with a wide range of professional colleagues.

Image Analysis and Interpretation

Fascinating, and highly promising, are the computer's growing powers of image analysis and interpretation. Computer-aided diagnosis (CAD) is in its infancy, yet computer-based expert systems, neural networks, and related tools are already playing important new roles in helping physicians make diagnoses. Of particular interest are computer programs adept at pattern recognition. Some have learned to analyze electrocardiograms (which you can think of as one-dimensional images) with success rates comparable to those of cardiologists, and they can do so for hours on end without growing the least bit bleary-eyed. The application of computers to two-dimensional images is far more challenging and will be slower in coming. But the writing is clearly on the wall-mounted, thin-panel liquid crystal display monitor.

Image processing, management, communication, and analysis in the clinic are likely to improve significantly in the near future. The technologies are being developed commercially, and powerful hardware and software tools produced for the military, the intelligence community, the space program, and the basic sciences are being transferred into the medical imaging research laboratories and clinics. It is not obvious where these developments will steer the field, but one thing is certain: the applications of computers in medical imaging will continue to evolve rapidly and to surprise us.

Wavelets Are Enhancing Medical Imaging

By Michael Unser, Akram Aldroubi, and Andrew Laine

Experts generally agree that the biggest advance in medical imaging in the last two decades of the twentieth century was the use of computers to assemble data from imaging devices into highly detailed pictures. Computed tomography, magnetic resonance imaging, and positron emission tomography all rely on computers to make sense of the data collected by the machines. To do so, computer programs increasingly depend on wavelets. These are mathematical tools, first developed in the early twentieth century, that allow wave data at various scales to be integrated into a whole. They have proven extremely useful in computerized medical imaging.

In the selection that follows three experts describe the boom in wavelet applications. In particular, they mention the usefulness of wavelets in screening out "noise"—the technical term for random perturbations on a signal. Wavelets also prove useful in tomography, the assembly of shots from multiple angles into a sectional image. Wavelets hold promise for helping radiologists detect signs of cancer in computer-aided mammography as well. The authors conclude that wavelets are integral to understanding wave data, such as that generated by imaging devices. Michael Unser is a professor of biomedical imaging at the Swiss Federal Institute of Technology, Lausanne. Akram Aldroubi is a professor of mathematics at Vanderbilt University. Andrew Laine is a professor of biomedical engineering at Columbia University.

Wavelets are the result of collective efforts that recognized common threads between ideas and concepts that had been independently developed and investigated by distinct research communities. They provide a unifying framework for decomposing images, volumes, and time series data into their elementary constituents across scale. Although a relatively recent construct, wavelets have become a tool of choice for engineers, physicists and mathematicians, leading to efficient solutions in time and space frequency analysis problems, as well as a multitude of other applications. One of the consequences is that wavelet methods of analysis and representation are presently having a significant impact on the science of medical imaging and the diagnosis of disease and screening protocols. Because of a powerful underlying mathematical theory, they offer exciting opportunities for the design of new multi-resolution image processing algorithms, and novel acquisition methods such as wavelet-encoded MRI. . . .

Rarely has a mathematical concept generated so much response and enthusiasm within and between the engineering and mathematical research communities at large. To give a rough idea of the phenomenon, we provide a brief chronology. While wavelets have been traced all the way back, to [Hungarian mathematician] Alfred Haar in 1910, for many, the starting point of their modern history coincides with two publications in the late 80s by [French mathematician] S. [Stéphane] Mallat and [Princeton University math professor] Ingrid Daubechies. These groundbreaking papers established a solid mathematical footing which would both shape and define the field. In a nutshell, S. Mallat identified the important concept of multiresolution analysis which is the corner stone of modern wavelet theory, while Ingrid Daubechies constructed the first orthogonal wavelet bases that were compactly supported. These two contributions count among the most cited papers in the scientific literature (over 1500 . . . citations each). From that point on, the number of contributions relating to wavelet-applications and theory has increased steadily on the order of 9000 journal papers published to date. . . .

Wavelets have become so popular that distinct, communities continue to have conferences and scientific journals entirely devoted to them. . . .

Given the size of the phenomenon, it is no suprise that wavelets have had an impact on a number of disciplines, medical imaging being no exception. A first record of activity in this particular area is the workshop on wavelets in medicine and biology that took place at the annual IEEE-EMBS [Institute of Electrical and Electronics Engineers-Engineering in Medicine and Biology Society] meeting, Baltimore, 1992. The first journal paper describing a wavelet application in medical imaging—noise reduction in MRI by soft-thresholding in the wavelet domain—also appeared in 1992. Note that this work, which is often overlooked, provides the earliest description of a wavelet denoising method that has become extremely popular. . . . So far, the primary applications of wavelets in medical imaging have been the following:

- Compression of medical images
- CT reconstruction; local tomography
- Wavelet denoising (MRI, ultrasound)
- Wavelet-based feature extraction; texture and statistical descriptors
- Medical image enhancement (e.g. fluoroscopy, mammography)
- Analysis of functional images of the brain (PET, IMRI)
- Wavelet-encoded MRI . . .

Functional imaging is an area were methods of wavelet processing hold great promise. This particular line of research was initiated by Urs Ruttimann, a creative researcher and good friend, who sadly passed away shortly before the publication of his paper in this very journal [*IEEE Transactions on Medical Imaging*]. Another first rate statistician who was also active in this area at an early stage is Jonathan Raz. By a sad coincidence, he also suffered a sudden death about a week before he was to present his latest results on wavelet analysis of functional magnetic resonance imaging (fMRI) . . .

Improving Mammograms

The recent development of commercial digital mammography imaging systems not only provides a significant improvement in image quality for traditional screening, but translates into a wealth of information for the analysis and detection of mammographic features by computer. . . . Papers by [Ghislain] Lemaur et al. and [Peter] Heinlein et al. focus on the goals of early detection and visual enhancement of microcalcifications, respectively. In the former, the regularity of a wavelet basis is used to identify microcalcification in clusters. The identification of microcalcifaction in clusters as opposed to individual occurrences is of clinical significance as clusters may suggest the likelihood of malignancy. In the later paper, a discretization of the continuous wavelet transform is a development which allows a filterbank to be adapted for the enhancement of mammographic features. This implementation allows for the reconstruction of modified wavelet coefficients at arbitrary scales and orientations without the introduction of artifacts or loss of completeness. The integration of such an interactive enhancement tool into digital mammographic screening systems will be of great importance as the wealth of dynamic range (contrast) provided by digital detectors become generally available to radiologists through the introduction of lower cost softcopy display systems. . . .

Careful Compression Needed

The amount of data generated by modern imaging devices is often very large, and ever increasing. Thus, an important problem is to find efficient ways of compressing and encoding this information to facilitate its transmission, storage, and retrieval. Since wavelet transforms provide sparse representations of signals, one of their privileged areas of application has been coding and compression. In fact, wavelets have had so much success in this area that they have already become an integral part of the new JPEG2000 [computer image] compression standard. Unlike other applications, however, biomedical image compression raises delicate issues; lossy compression must be done carefully so as to preserve all medically relevant information while eventually suppressing irrelevant features such as noise or background. Thus, research in this area must address these specific needs and pay great attention to the issue of validation. . . .

After having completed tasks of putting this [selection] together and based on our collective knowledge in the field, it is our belief that wavelets are here to stay. The idea of decomposing a signal according to scale is as fundamental a notion for imaging as decomposing it into harmonic components (Fourier analysis); it is more intuitive and closer to what the visual system does. Another important point that has stimulated wavelet research is the quest for sparse representations of signals, as these offer obvious advantages for data compression, noise reduction and regularization purposes. As more progress is made in the years ahead, it is quite possible that the importance of wavelets as a research topic in its own right may diminish and that they will progressively reach the status of standard toolbox components for data processing (such as the FFT). Indeed, we are seeing some of this maturity in the development of emerging commercial image analysis software and packages. Yet, given the flexibility of this powerful analysis tool, there is not much risk in betting that wavelets will continue to be widely used in a diversity of medical imaging applications.

A beneficial side effect of all the interdisciplinary activity taking place around wavelets has been to create a common language between mathematicians and engineers and to instill rigor in the formulation of imaging problems. Wavelets have been a cross-cutting magnet encouraging engineers to use more sophisticated mathematics and mathematicians to consider applying their knowledge to real world problems.

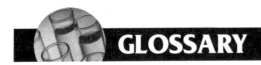

GLOSSARY

angiocardiography: X-ray imaging of the heart and the major blood vessels around it. The organs are made visible by the injection of a special X-ray absorbing agent. (See contrast medium.)

angiography: an X-ray technique that uses injected X-ray-blocking dye to enhance the imaging of the major arteries and veins of the neck and brain. It is used to identify narrowing of the arteries as well as aneurysms and vascular malformations.

arthrography: an X-ray examination of joints, especially the knee, often involving the injection of dyes or other contrast materials to enhance the image.

computed tomography: often known as a CT or CAT scan, this is a technique in which multiple X-ray "slice" images through the body are combined by a computer to obtain a highly detailed cross-sectional image.

contrast medium (CM): a dense or radioactive substance that the patient ingests to heighten the contrast in a medical image. Typically, a contrast medium is needed to image an internal organ because the tissue is insufficiently dense to absorb enough X-rays to show up.

diagnostic ultrasound: see ultrasound.

digital radiography: a technology that captures X-ray images without film. A fluorescent plate reacts to the X-rays and is scanned by a laser imaging system. The system then converts the lighter and darker sections into pixels that are digitally encoded in a computer to be reconstructed as an image.

Doppler effect: an apparent change in frequency of a wave caused by motion toward or away from the source, as when the pitch of a train whistle seems to drop as it passes by a stationary listener.

Doppler ultrasound: a sophisticated ultrasound scanner that makes use of the Doppler effect to determine the velocity and direction of blood flow or other bodily fluids. (See Doppler effect.)

dynamic imaging: the recording of flow, pooling, or uptake of a substance to create sequential images of internal bodily functions. For example, the flow of blood through the aorta, highlighted by a contrast agent, might be used to record the functioning of the heart. (See also functional MRI.)

electroencephalogram (EEG): a graphic record of electrical activity in the brain as detected by electrodes placed on the skull.

endoscopy: the imaging of internal organs by means of fiber-optic instruments inserted through an orifice. Endoscopy is an invasive form of medical imaging.

fluoroscope: a device equipped with a fluorescent screen that glows when X-rays, passing through an optically opaque object such as the human body, strike the screen. The contrast between brighter and darker glowing areas creates a real-time, moving image. Fluoroscopes were widely used in shoe stores and medical clinics before the dangers of continuous exposure to X-rays were understood.

functional MRI (fMRI): a variant of magnetic resonance imaging that captures sequential images of blood flow in the brain, showing how the brain functions. The technology is based on the understanding that the active regions of the brain need more blood than the inactive ones. In some cases short movies, called "cines," can be made. (See also magnetic resonance imaging.)

gamma rays: high-energy electromagnetic rays, or photons, emitted by radioactive isotopes. In nuclear medicine these are typically the photons emitted from the body that special cameras pick up and turn into images.

ionizing radiation: high-energy electromagnetic radiation, such as X-rays, that has the capability of causing molecules or atoms to become electrically charged variants called ions. This process of ionization can damage DNA, potentially leading to cancer.

magnetic resonance imaging (MRI): a noninvasive imaging technique that uses a powerful magnetic field to align atoms within the body and then disturb them with a pulse of radiowaves. The resulting radiowave echoes are recorded by the MRI machine and computed to form an image.

mammogram: a mammary image produced by flattening the breast and then X-raying it in search of cancerous growths.

mammography: imaging of the breast by means of X-rays, ultrasound, or other means to screen for breast disease. (See mammogram.)

nuclear imaging: imaging techniques that involve the use of a radioactive isotope targeted at an area of interest in the patient's body. After the radioactive substance is injected or inhaled, it collects in the area of interest, and the imaging device captures high-energy photons that the isotope gives off and uses them to compose an image. (See also positron-emission tomography and single photon emission computed tomography.)

positron-emission tomography (PET): a method of nuclear imaging that relies on positrons—the positive version of electrons—to create flashes of electromagnetic energy, which can be recorded and turned into an image. When a positron encounters an electron in the body, they mutually annihilate, turning into gamma rays that are detected outside the body and processed into images. Positron-bearing isotopes are generated in a special machine called a cyclotron and injected into the patient at the time of the examination.

radiography: the imaging of any part of the body for diagnostic purposes by means of X-rays. The image may be captured on film, observed in fluorescence, or turned directly into digital data.

radiologic technologists (RTs): technicians who are trained to perform diagnostic imaging examinations and administer radiation therapy treatments. They are educated in anatomy, patient positioning, examination techniques, equipment protocols, radiation safety, radiation protection, and basic patient care.

radiologist: a physician who specializes in medical imaging, including X-ray technology, magnetic resonance imaging, and ultrasound diagnosis.

radionuclide: a radioactive isotope used in certain medical imaging procedures. The medically useful radionuclides are radioactive for a relatively short period, ranging from hours to days, so as to make imaging possible without endangering the patient.

single photon emission computed tomography (SPECT): a nuclear imaging technique that relies on a radionuclide circulating in the blood to give off gamma rays. A camera or multiple cameras rotating around the patient pick up gamma ray photons, and a computer assembles them into a three-dimensional image.

technetium-99m (99mTc): a radionuclide widely used in nuclear imaging. With a half life of just six hours, technetium-99m poses little danger to the patient. It also binds well with various carrier molecules that can be targeted to specific tissues. (See also nuclear imaging and radionuclide.)

ultrasound: an imaging technique involving the use of extremely high-frequency sound waves to penetrate the body and then bounce back to the surface, where the echoes can be captured and converted into images of the structures within the body.

X-ray: a form of electromagnetic radiation (like visible light, only of much higher frequency) that can penetrate ordinary matter. Discovered by Wilhelm C. Röntgen in 1895, X-rays can be generated by directing powerful electron beams at a target that reacts by emitting high-energy photons. The slight absorption of X-rays by flesh and bone allows for images of internal bodily structures.

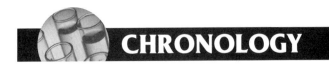

CHRONOLOGY

A.D. 130

Greek physician Galen is born. He describes (inaccurately) the interior of the human body. Galen's writings become the foundation of Western medicine for more than a millenium.

1537

Anatomist Andreas Vesalius begins making accurate anatomical sketches based on the dissection of executed criminals.

1564

Galileo Galilei is born. He is a pathfinding scientist who is credited with putting the study of acoustics on a modern scientific footing.

1822

Swiss physicist Daniel Colladen uses an underwater bell to estimate the speed of sound in the waters of Lake Geneva. Understanding the variable speed of sound through different media creates the basis for ultrasound imaging.

1859

Physicist Julius Plucker identifies cathode rays (electron streams in a tube), a preliminary step on the way to the discovery of X-rays.

1878

William Crookes of Britain creates the prototype cathode ray tube (CRT), forerunner of the modem television tube, and accidentally creates X-rays but fails to understand what they are.

1895

Wilhelm C. Röntgen of Germany, following up on the experiments of Crookes and others, discovers X-rays and uses them to produce the first medical X-ray image (of his wife's hand).

1897

Italy becomes the first nation to use X-rays in battlefield hospitals.

1898

The U.S. Army uses X-rays for the first time to assist military surgeons during Spanish-American War.

1901

Röntgen receives a Nobel Prize for his discovery.

1904

The first death attributed to overexposure to X-rays occurs. The victim was a glassblower working in Thomas Edison's lab.

1905

Elizabeth Aschein becomes the first X-ray technician to die from radiation exposure after working twelve-hour days for many years without protection.

1913

An improved X-ray generation tube replaces the Crookes tube.

1917

French physicist Paul Langevin opens the era of ultrasonics with the invention of high-frequency acoustic sonar for submarine detection.

1920

X-ray fluoroscopes go into wide use in medical clinics and other arenas, including shoe stores.

1932

Physicist Carl Anderson discovers the positron, later to be used as the basis for positron-emission tomography.

1937

Physicist Isidor Rabi observes nuclear magnetic resonance (NMR), the basis for magnetic resonance imaging.

1942

Researcher Karl Dussik of Austria publishes the first paper on the medical potential of ultrasonics, based on flawed but promising attempts to image the brain with ultrasound.

1944

Rabi receives the Nobel Prize for his discovery of NMR.

1946

Physicists Felix Bloch and Edward Purcell demonstrate that magnetic resonance can identify every type of atomic nucleus.

1950

Massachusetts Institute of Technology (MIT) opens an acoustics lab dedicated to researching the use of ultrasound for diagnosis. Medical researcher Gordon Brownell conducts the first imaging experiment using positron emissions at the Physics Research Laboratory of Massachusetts General Hospital.

1952

First positron-emission scan image is obtained. It is a crude series of marks projected onto a sketch of a head.

1953

The American Institute of Ultrasound in Medicine (AIUM) holds its first scientific meeting.

1959

Professor Ian Donald of Scotland detects a fetus's head in the womb using ultrasound.

1965

First International Conference on Diagnostic Ultrasound is held in Pittsburgh, as ultrasound scanners go into wide clinical use.

1969

The First World Congress on Ultrasonic Diagnostics in Medicine is held in Vienna.

1971

Physician and medical researcher Raymond Damadian publishes a paper on alleged variations in the magnetic resonance of malignant and healthy rat tissues.

1972

British engineer Godfrey Hounsfield performs the first X-ray-computed axial tomography scan. Gordon Brownell, David Chesler, and colleagues produce positron-emission tomography (PET) images.

1973

Chemistry professor Paul Lauterbur publishes the first MRI image, taken of two water-filled tubes. Mathematician Peter Mansfield lays the groundwork for the development of high-speed and detailed magnetic resonance images through use of gradients (variations in magnetic fields). Chemists Edward J. Hoffman and Michael Phelps develop the first human PET scanner at Washington University in St. Louis.

1974

Damadian receives a patent for an MRI cancer-detection device. Swiss scientist Richard Ernst of Switzerland creates a method for applying mathematical tools called Fourier transforms to swiftly convert the raw data from an MRI into a viewable image. Electrical engineer Donald Baker and colleagues create a Doppler ultrasound scanner capable of tracking blood flow.

1975

Mansfield shows how to use radio pulses in MRI to produce high-resolution images.

1976

Computed tomography X-ray scanners capable of imaging any part of the human body become available.

1977

Damadian produces the first MRI image of a human body.

1979

Hounsfield and Allen Cormack share a Nobel Prize for having launched computed tomography in 1972.

1981

The first commercial MRI scanner goes into operation.

1984

Increased computing power allows for development of three-dimensional images from CT or MRI scans.

1989

Spiral CT X-ray scanning debuts, greatly speeding the process of capturing computed tomography images.

1991

Ernst receives the Nobel Prize for his contributions to gaining high resolution in nuclear magnetic resonance spectroscopy.

1993

Echo planar magnetic resonance imaging is introduced to provide early detection of strokes. Also known as functional MRI, this technology allows researchers to observe the brain in action.

2000

First digital mammography unit gains Food and Drug Administration approval.

2003

The Nobel Prize in Medicine goes to Lauterbur and Mansfield for the development of imaging techniques using magnetic resonance. Damadian vigorously objects to their recognition.

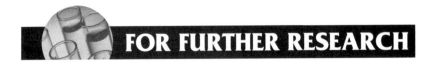
FOR FURTHER RESEARCH

Books

Mark A. Brown and Richard C. Semelka, *MRI: Basic Principles and Applications.* New York: Wiley-Liss, 1995.

Stewart C. Bushong, *Computed Tomography.* New York: McGraw-Hill, 2000.

Richard B. Buxton, *Introduction to Functional Magnetic Resonance Imaging: Principles and Techniques.* New York: Cambridge University Press, 2002.

Roberto Cabeza and Alan Kingstone, eds., *Handbook of Functional Neuroimaging of Cognition.* Cambridge, MA: MIT Press, 2001.

Paul T. Callaghan, *Principles of Nuclear Magnetic Resonance Microscopy.* New York: Oxford University Press, 1991.

Lisa Cartwright, *Screening the Body: Tracing Medicine's Visual Culture.* Minneapolis: University of Minnesota Press, 1995.

Committee on Technologies for the Early Detection of Breast Cancer, *Mammography and Beyond: Developing Technologies for the Early Detection of Breast Cancer.* Washington, DC: National Academy, 2001.

Lachlan De Crespigny, *Which Tests for My Unborn Baby? Ultrasound and Other Prenatal Tests.* New York: Oxford University Press, 1996.

E. Gordon DePuey, Daniel S. Berman, and Ernest V. Garcia, eds., *Cardiac SPECT Imaging.* New York: Raven, 1995.

Ronald L. Eisenberg, *Radiology: An Illustrated History.* Saint Louis, MO: Mosby, 1992.

P.J. Ell and B.L. Holman, eds., *Computed Emission Tomography.* Oxford, UK: Oxford University Press, 1982.

William A. Ewing, *Inside Information: Imaging the Human Body.* New York: Simon & Schuster, 1996.

Terri L. Fauber, *Radiographic Imaging and Exposure.* St. Louis, MO: Mosby, 2000.

Ray Freeman, *Magnetic Resonance in Chemistry and Medicine.* New York: Oxford University Press, 2003.

Ray H. Hashemi and William G. Bradley Jr., *MRI: The Basics.* Baltimore: Williams & Wilkins, 1997.

Peter Jezzard, Paul M. Matthews, and Stephen M. Smith, eds., *Functional MRI: An Introduction to Methods.* New York: Oxford University Press, 2001.

Willi A. Kalender, *Computed Tomography: Fundamentals, System Technology, Image Quality, Applications.* Indianapolis: Wiley, 2005.

Bettyann Kevles, *Naked to the Bone: Medical Imaging in the Twentieth Century.* New Brunswick, NJ: Rutgers University Press, 1997.

Frederick W. Kremkau, *Doppler Ultrasound: Principles and Instruments.* Philadelphia: W.B. Saunders, 1990.

Vadim Kuperman, *Magnetic Resonance Imaging: Physical Principles and Applications.* San Diego: Academic Press, 2000.

Albert Macovski, *Medical Imaging Systems.* Englewood Cliffs, NJ: Prentice-Hall, 1983.

James Mattson, *The Pioneers of NMR and Magnetic Resonance in Medicine: The Story of MRI.* Jericho, NY: Dean, 1996.

Kendall Preston Jr., ed., *Medical Imaging Techniques: A Comparison.* New York: Plenum, 1979.

Sunder S. Rajan, *MRI: A Conceptual Overview.* New York: Springer, 1998.

Helen C. Redman and Allan E. Fisch, *Computed Tomography of the Body.* Philadelphia: Saunders, 1979.

Carol M. Rumack, Stephanie R. Wilson, and J. William Charboneau, eds., *Diagnostic Ultrasound.* 2nd ed. Saint Louis, MO: Mosby, 1998.

F.A. Smith, *A Primer in Applied Radiation Physics.* River Edge, NJ: World Scientific, 2000.

Perry Sprawls Jr., *Physical Principles of Medical Imaging.* Rockville, MD: Aspen, 1987.

Nora D. Volkow and Alfred P. Wolf, eds., *Positron-Emission Tomography in Schizophrenia Research.* Washington, DC: American Psychiatric Press, 1991.

Anthony Brinton Wolbarst, *Looking Within: How X-ray, CT, MRI, Ultrasound, and Other Medical Images Are Created, and How They Help Physicians Save Lives.* Berkeley: University of California Press, 1999.

Periodicals

Gary Chamberlain, "Medical Images to Move on the Internet Using Java," *Design News*, March 1, 1999.

Mark Fischetti, "Working Knowledge," *Scientific American*, August 2004.

Carol Gentry, "Seeing the Body Electric, in 3-D," *Wall Street Journal*, January 24, 2000.

Anne Harding, "New Breast Imaging Detects Smallest Tumors," Reuters, January 20, 2005. www.nlm.nih.gov.

Jenny Hogan, "Imaging Thin Air Can Spot Lung Disease," *New Scientist*, April 10, 2004.

Karen Houppert, "Would You Want to See Your Unborn Baby in 3-D?" *Self*, August 2000.

Hassaun Jones-Bey, "The Dilemma of Medical Screening," *Laser Focus World*, May 2000.

Olga Kharif, "Focusing on Picture-Perfect Diagnoses," *Business Week Online*, October 17, 2002. www.businessweek.com.

Gina Kolata, "Rapid Rise and Fall for Body-Scanning Clinics," *New York Times*, January 23, 2005.

David C. Levin, "Me and My MRI," *New York Times*, July 6, 2004.

Corie Lok, "Picture Perfect," *Nature*, July 26, 2001.

Lucas Mearian, "Medical Imaging Strains Storage," *Computerworld*, September 3, 2001.

Norman B. Medow, "Modern Imaging Techniques Driven by Past Pioneers," *Ophthalmology Times*, July 15, 2001.

Kenneth J. Nazintsky and Burton M. Gold, "Radiology—Then and Now," *American Journal of Roentgenology*, August 1988.

Jason Ocker, "MRI 'Excellent Choice' for Overcoming Challenges of Diagnosing Pregnant Women with Abdominal Pain," *Medical News Today*, February 3, 2005.

Michael E. Phelps and John C. Mazziotta, "Positron Emission Tomography: Human Brain Function and Biochemistry," *Science*, May 17, 1985.

Judith E. Randall, "NMR: The Best Thing Since X-Rays?" *Technology Review*, January 1988.

Rhonda Rundle, "In Stores Now: Full-Body Scans," *Wall Street Journal*, July 24, 2001.

———, "PET Scanners Become New Rx for Diagnostics," *Wall Street Journal*, May 6, 2003.

Judy Siegel-Itzkovich, "Fly's-Eye View Shines a Light on Disease," *New Scientist*, January 10, 2004.

Alexandra Stikeman, "Precision Brain Scans," *Technology Review*, October 2002.

Nathan Stormer, "Seeing the Fetus: The Role of Technology and Image in the Maternal-Fetal Relationship," *Journal of the American Medical Association*, April 2, 2003.

Betsy Streisand, "Profiting from Patient Paranoia?" *U.S. News & World Report*, June 7, 1999.

Sterling Thomas, "Computers and Cancer, *World & I*, March 2004.

R.L. Wahl, "Positron Emission Tomography (PET): An Update on Applications in Breast Cancer," *Breast Disease*, October 1998.

Richard L. Weisfield, "Digital X-ray Imagers Fill Medical and NDT Tasks," *Laser Focus World*, May 1999.

Anthony B. Wolbarst, "Full-Body CT Scans: Too Much Radiation? Study Finds High Potential Doses, but Other Scan Dangers Likely Worse," American Cancer Society, September 3, 2004. www.cancer.org.

————, "Tune in to Terahertz," *Economist*, August 10, 2002.

Roisin Woolnough, "Heart of the Matter," *Computer Weekly*, June 20, 2002.

Web Sites

American Cancer Society, www.cancer.org. This is a nationwide, community-based health organization dedicated to the fight against cancer. Site includes an overview of medical imaging techniques under the "Prevention and Early Detection" section.

American College of Radiology, www.acr.org. This is the site of the leading national organization for radiologists. It includes a news page and a searchable database of radiology-related information.

American Heart Association (AHA), www.americanheart.org. The AHA is a national voluntary health agency whose mission is to reduce disability and death from cardiovascular diseases and stroke. Included on the site is information about MRI for the heart.

American Society of Echocardiography, www.asecho.org. The society represents cardiac ultrasound specialists. Its site includes a patient information page at www.seemyheart.org.

American Society of Radiologic Technologists, www.asrt.org. This organization represents more than one hundred thousand skilled operators of medical imaging devices. Its site includes pages for the public.

Mayo Clinic, www.mayoclinic.com. Operated by the Mayo Foundation for Medical Education and Research, this site provides a large array of medical information pages, including many on medical imaging.

Radiological Society of North America (RSNA), www.radiology info.org. The RSNA is an association of more than thirty-five thousand radiologists, radiation oncologists, and related scientists committed to promoting excellence in radiology. Their site offers pages explaining many forms of medical imaging.

U.S. Food and Drug Administration (FDA), www.fda.gov. This is the federal agency that regulates medical imaging. Its site includes *FDA Consumer*, a magazine with occasional articles on medical imaging, and news alerts, as well as general information.

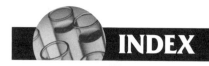

INDEX